Hotel, Hostel and Hospital Housekeeping

Joan C. Branson

B.Sc., M.H.C.I.M.A.,
Lecturer, The School of Hotel Keeping and Catering,
Ealing Technical College

Margaret Lennox

DIP. DOM. SCI.,
Formerly Lecturer, Department of Hotel and Catering Management
University of Surrey, Formerly Battersea College of Technology

Incorporating the Second Edition (Metric) of
Hotel Housekeeping

Edward Arnold

© Joan C. Branson and Margaret Lennox 1976

First published 1965
by Edward Arnold (Publishers) Ltd.,
25 Hill Street, London, W1X 8LL

Reprinted 1967
Second Edition (Metric) 1971
Reprinted 1972, 1973

Third Edition 1976

ISBN: 0 7131 1974 8

Printed and bound in Canada by The Hunter Rose Co., Toronto, Ontario.

Introduction to the Third Edition

The planning, provision and service of accommodation in hotels, hostels, hospitals and similar establishments is a task involving many thousands of people and many thousands of pounds in its operation.

The management of the housekeeping department, particularly in some spheres, has advanced rapidly in recent years and requires not only a knowledge of technical skills but also an understanding of the 'tools' of management. A large part of the executive housekeeper's time is taken up with personnel management and her aim should be an efficiently run department with as low operating costs as possible. Her work involves providing a clean, comfortable and safe environment, and a well organised department should contribute significantly to the profitability of the establishment. The housekeeping department should not be considered in isolation as it is an important source of information for many other departments and good co-operation leads to a more congenial atmosphere throughout the establishment.

In this book the above aspects of housekeeping have been explained and it is hoped that they meet the needs of students and anyone interested in this field of study. The context and structure of the book have been influenced by the requirements of the various examining bodies in the Hotel and Catering field.

It is not expected that the book will be read at one sitting, therefore some degree of repetition has been introduced where it is considered necessary, and cross-references have been provided in order to ensure a comprehensive understanding of each chapter.

J.C.B.
M.L.

Metrication

Throughout this edition imperial measurements have been replaced by metric units. This includes the use of the degree Celsius. Only on one or two occasions where sizes are still thought of in imperial terms (e.g. beds) have we included the equivalents. The following brief table gives conversions for the quantities most often referred to in the book:

1 inch	= 2.54 cm
1 foot	= 30.48 cm
1 square inch	= 6.45 cm²
1 square foot	= 929.03 cm² = 0.0929 m²
1 pound	= 0.454 kg
1 pint	= 0.568 litres
1 dwt (24 grains)	= 1.555 grammes (g)

Acknowledgements

Without help and encouragement this book would not have been written and we are fortunate in that many hotels, hospitals, hostels and university halls of residence, far too numerous to mention all by name, have opened their doors to us in our quest for information.

We are greatly indebted to the staff of the Hotel and Catering departments of our respective Colleges for their helpful advice and criticism and we appreciate the help our respective families have afforded us, as well as their unfailing interest.

The publishers wish to thank the following for permission to reproduce copyright photographs:
Antiference Curtain Rails 123, 124; Architectural Review 206; Austin Suite Ltd 219 btm; Barnaby's Picture Library 226; Brecht-Einzig Ltd 206; British Red Cross 245, 246; Buckingham Beds 178 top; Concord Lighting Co Ltd 205 top right, 206 btm; Doulton Sanitaryware 225; Flexello Ltd 191; Flowers and Plants Council 211; Formica Ltd 219 top, 223; Garnett College 229, 231; Heals Contracts Ltd 185 top right; Heathrow Hotel 93, 94; Hoover Ltd 21, 22; Inn on the Park 121, 152, 205 top left, btm right, 224; Johnson Wax 24; Noeline Kelly 20, 25, 47, 51, 57, 77, 79, 81, 93, 94, 120 btm, 127, 132, 152, 171, 176, 177, 178 btm, 185 top left, 188 top left, btm right, 208, 218, 221, 229; Marks and Spencer Ltd 186; MAS Contracts Ltd 180 c; Parker-Knoll Ltd 188 top right; Primo Furniture Ltd 180 btm right, 185 top left, 192; Royal Garden Hotel 51, 79, 81, 178 btm, 205 btm left, 208, 218, 221; Royal Kensington Hotel 47, 132, 188 btm; Rufflette Ltd 120 top, 121; Selfridges Ltd 127, 171, 177, 185, 188 top left; Julie Stevens 180 d, 248; Stilsound Blinds Ltd 125; Tower Hotel 20, 25, 57, 77, 176, 207; Victoria and Albert Museum 180 a, b; Vitopan Ltd 23.

Contents

1

The Housekeeper and her Staff

Housekeeping or domestic administration is essential in all types of establishments be they hotels, clubs, hospitals or hostels in order that there shall be comfort, cleanliness and service, and all these should be the concern of every member of the establishment.

The responsibility for housekeeping is usually that of a woman but in some cases it is undertaken by a man, for example a college bursar, a restaurant manager or a hospital administrator, and even where it is that of a woman the exact title of the person may vary from one establishment to another. In hostels and university halls of residence domestic bursars may be engaged, one of whom is responsible for the housekeeping but where the welfare of the residents comes within the scope of the person, the term warden is more usual. In the case of hospitals, domestic manager or domestic superintendent may be the title or even warden of a nurses' home. Matron is often used in homes for old people and children, and in boarding schools.

In hotels, housekeeper is the usual title, but there are hotels where the manageress may in fact be the housekeeper although she would obviously prefer to be known as manageress since this infers a higher status.

It is one thing to give the correct title to the person responsible for housekeeping in a particular establishment, but it is quite another matter to find a suitable title when referring to establishments in general. 'House services' manager' or 'Controller of house services' are possible terms but throughout this book the appropriate titles will be used where possible and where this is not so, the term *housekeeper* will be used, irrespective of the type or size of the establishment or house.

A similar problem arises with regard to the word guest/resident/patient/customer, etc., and so again the appropriate word will be used where possible, otherwise the word *guest* will be used generally.

The management of the housekeeping department will be influenced by such factors as size, type and location of the establishment and no two *housekeepers* will manage their departments in exactly the same way. However, whether the department is large or small, luxury or medium class, for short or long stays, from the commercial or welfare field, management expects the department to be run with the highest degree of efficiency and at the lowest cost.

The standard and tone of the housekeeping department plays a large part in the reputation of the establishment and in determining whether *guests* are happy during their stay, and in the case of hotels, wish to return. Whereas the type of service offered differs greatly from one establishment to another and as a result housekeeping in hotels and expensive clubs may be more specialised than in other establishments, the basic problems of administration are similar. Efficiency in house-keeping should lead to the comfort and well-being of the *guest*, and this in hotels, clubs and hostels should lead to a greater or full occupancy and in hospitals the patient should leave satisfied that as well as medical and nursing care, his comfort had been considered. Besides this, efficiency in housekeeping should contribute to the saving in costs of labour, cleaning materials and equipment, furnishings and the like in every type of establishment.

The *housekeeper* who has the ability and personality to make *guests* feel welcome, to inspire confidence, to smooth over difficulties and to train her staff is an asset in any establishment and should save management many headaches.

A housekeeper's work may consist of some or all of the following:

Co-operation with other departments;
Engagement, dismissal and welfare of her staff;
Supervision, control and training of her staff;
Compilation of duty rosters, holiday lists and wage sheets;
Checking the cleanliness of offices, lounges, guest and staff rooms;
Completion and/or checking of room occupancy lists;
Dealing with guests' complaints and requests;
Reporting and checking of all maintenance work;
Control and supervision of the work of the linen room and possibly the laundry;
Dealing with lost property;
Responsibility for the keys in her department;
Prevention of fire and other accidents in her department;
Care of the sick and the provision of First Aid for staff and guests;
Ordering and issuing of stores in her department;
Keeping inventories and records of equipment, redecoration and any other relevant details of the department;
Responsibility for the floral decorations.

When considering a housekeeping department it must be realised that there are different types of establishments, that many variations within one type will exist and that, however similar, no two places will be run exactly alike. Classification is therefore difficult.

Very broadly, the establishments may be classified as welfare or commercial. In the former category are hostels and homes of various kinds, university halls of residence, boarding schools and hospitals and in the latter, hotels of various kinds, motels, expensive clubs, private nursing homes, holiday camps and boarding houses.

In the welfare or non-commercial field a reasonable standard of cleanliness, comfort and service is expected at the lowest possible cost, irrespective of the size of the establishment. With this end in view, in many university halls of residence, hostels for young people, old people's homes, etc., residents may be expected to make their own beds and do other small jobs. In some instances laundering and cooking facilities may be provided for the use of the residents.

In boarding schools there may be a number of single or double study bedrooms, but there will, in addition, be larger areas, e.g. dormitories and classrooms, to be looked after. Furnishings are normally kept very simple.

In hospitals, the staff residences may be likened to halls of residence. Hospitals contain administrative areas, laboratories, training schools, laundries, kitchens and staff residences as well as patient areas. In the patient areas there must be emphasis on the control of infection.

In many of these establishments the *housekeeper* will have one or more assistants working for her. The assistants will supervise those undertaking the actual cleaning and carry out work delegated to them by the *housekeeper*. In these establishments there may be individual names for maids carrying out specific jobs, e.g. ward orderlies, ward maids, but in most cases those who do the actual cleaning are called 'maids', 'domestic assistants' or 'cleaners' without any reference to the location of their work.

HOSPITALS

In hospitals the staffing structure is different from other establishments and the names of certain grades may be found confusing (e.g. senior housekeepers in hospitals are not the highest grade).

The District Domestic Services Manager is responsible for the domestic services in a group of hospitals and he or she has working for him:

Domestic Superintendents who will be responsible for the day-to-day organisation of the domestic services of one of the larger or several of the smaller hospitals within the group.

Assistant Domestic Superintendents may be in sole charge of the domestic services of a small hospital (perhaps 130 beds) or will undertake some of the work of the Domestic Superintendent in a larger hospital.

Senior Housekeepers may be in sole charge of the domestic services of

DISTRICT DOMESTIC SERVICES MANAGER

Hospital (a) 205 beds acute	Hospital (b) 261 acute	Hospital (c) 81 beds orthopaedic	Hospital (d) 130 beds children	Hospital (e) 740 beds Mental Handicap	Hospital (f) 713 beds Geriatric
Domestic Superintendent	Domestic Superintendent			Domestic Superintendent	Domestic Superintendent
Assistant Domestic Superintendent	Assistant Domestic Superintendent		Assistant Domestic Superintendent	2 Assistant Domestic Superintendents	2 Assistant Domestic Superintendents
					Assistant Domestic Superintendent (Training)
3 Senior Housekeepers	Senior Housekeeper				

DOMESTIC SUPERVISORS
WARD HOUSEKEEPERS

DOMESTIC ASSISTANTS — WARD ORDERLIES
HOUSEKEEPING AIDS etc.

Typical organisation chart of the domestic services of the hospital division of a Health District a smaller hospital (80–120 beds) or may look after the domestic services of a similar number of beds in a larger hospital.

Domestic Supervisors are responsible for the day-to-day programme of cleaning work in the specific area allocated to them. They may be in charge of 20–25 domestic staff.

Domestic Assistants—Ward Orderlies—Housekeeping Aids are frequently part-time and their duties will depend on the particular areas in which they work, e.g. cleaning rooms, wards and related areas, departments, residences, washing-up, and special work such as floor cleaning.

The District Domestic Manager's duties will include:

Co-ordination, direction and control of the work of the staff in day-to-day control of the domestic services in each unit to ensure
    work schedules are drawn up;
    staffing levels are maintained;
    an acceptable standard of cleanliness is achieved and maintained in
        all parts of each hospital;
Organisation and supervision of training programmes;
Constant review of cleaning procedures;
Advice to the employing authority on
    level of expenditure;
    staffing requirements;
    planning of domestic services in relation to the support they are
        required to give to the nursing staff;
    cleaning policies in new buildings within the District;
Maintenance of such records as are necessary.

HOSTELS

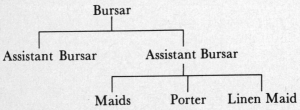

Organisation chart of a students' hostel

The Bursar (who is often a man) or a **Domestic Bursar** (who is a woman) is responsible for the management of the hostel, including the catering, housekeeping and maintenance of the building and grounds. There may also be a warden who will normally combine an academic post with that of being responsible for the welfare and discipline of the residents.

The Bursar is responsible for:

Assistant bursars, one or more of whom will supervise the maids and undertake the day-to-day running of the housekeeping department.

Maids/cleaners/domestic assistants who very frequently are part-time and do the work assigned to them by the assistant bursars.

Porters/male domestics, who do the heavier and dirtier work of the house and any other odd jobs.

Linen maid who looks after the work of the linen room.

Window cleaning is normally done on contract, but it may be done by the porters.

On a university campus there may be a number of halls of residence which from the administrative point of view are dealt with as one. Terminology of staff varies from one university to another and the following is a specific example of one university.

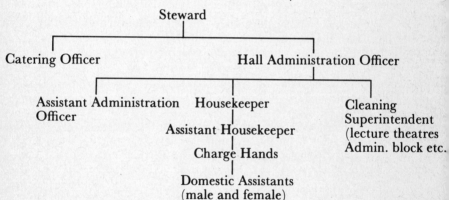

Organisation chart of one specific university

HOTELS

In the commercial field, guests are charged according to the type of accommodation and service they are offered. It is rather easier therefore to classify these establishments. Thus hotels and motels may be classified:

1   First-class luxury hotels with private bathrooms, suites and lounges, where the décor is luxurious and provision is made for particular personal services to the guests. This type of hotel will inevitably be very expensive and employ many staff, and there are only a few such hotels in this country.

2   Good hotels having private bathrooms, some suites, lounges, good décor, very comfortable but giving less personal service and so less expensive.

3   Medium-class hotels where comfort and furnishings are adequate but personal service is cut to a minimum and thus these hotels will be cheaper.

4   Small hotels with less than 50 bedrooms, where the furnishings and tariff vary tremendously. In such hotels the manager and his wife may manage with a general assistant and few other staff. Some or all staff may combine jobs, as for example the chambermaid may be a relief waitress and the houseporter may serve early morning tea, and thus this type of hotel is not an easy one to deal with as far as teaching is concerned but is by far the largest group in this country.

5   Motels, Post Houses and Motor hotels are specialised establishments catering for motorists, situated on a main trunk road. Fewer staff are employed and more 'do-it-yourself' equipment is found. Motels usually have parking facilities close by the accommodation.

Expensive clubs in town or country providing facilities for recreation and relaxation with some sleeping accommodation are run very much on the lines of a first-class hotel.

Holiday camps generally consist of chalet-type accommodation and the amount of service varies. In some places cooking facilities are provided for the guests.

Boarding houses are small hotels, generally with simple furnishings and providing little service.

According to the Catering Wages Order a head housekeeper in an hotel is one who supervises three or more assistant housekeepers. There are hotels where the head housekeeper is an executive housekeeper. The housekeeper in large hotels may be responsible for the following members of staff:

Assistant housekeepers (floor housekeepers or floor supervisors) who supervise the maids and carry out work delegated by the housekeeper.

Room-maids who are responsible for the servicing of the guests' bedrooms, private sitting rooms and often private bathrooms, and who are on call for service to guests.

Staff maids who clean the rooms of the living-in staff.

Cleaners who are usually part-time and whose job it is to clean offices, public rooms, bathrooms and ladies' cloakrooms. This work in some hotels may still be done by full-time housemaids or corridor maids, but owing to the difficulty of obtaining such maids these days, part-time cleaners have taken their place. There are firms which undertake contract cleaning and some hotels use this service, but the housekeeper still 'vets' their work.

Linen keeper who supervises the work of the linen room and who may have several linen maids to assist her in providing clean, presentable linen throughout the house.

Cloakroom attendant who looks after the ladies' powder room.

Houseporters whose work consists of the removal of rubbish, the shifting of furniture, heavy vacuum cleaning and other odd jobs.

Valet porters who usually only work in first-class hotels and are responsible for the valeting of the clothes of the male guests and combine this with some of the less dirty jobs of the houseporter (a full-time valet is not normally on the housekeeping staff).

A florist may be on the housekeeping staff, but in some hotels the housekeeper or her assistants may arrange the flowers, yet in others there may be contract arrangements.

Window-cleaning may be done on contract or by the houseporters.

In small hotels there may be a **General Assistant** who is expected to work in any department at any job.

In most hotels it is usual for the manager to confer with his heads of departments regarding day-to-day matters. His understanding of the work of each department is helpful for all concerned. He should inform the housekeeper of alterations or arrangements which may affect the running of her department, and she should inform him of any disturbances or unusual occurrences created by guests in their rooms.

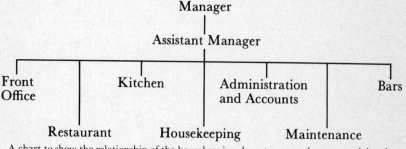

A chart to show the relationship of the housekeeping department to the managerial and other departments of the hotel

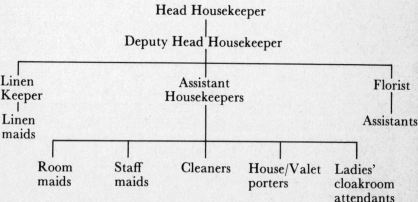

An organisation chart of a typical housekeeping department in a large hotel

Co-operation

In all establishments during the course of her work the *housekeeper* comes in contact with the staff responsible for other parts of the establishment and for smooth running there must be close interdepartmental co-operation. Depending on the type and size of the house, the work in each of the other departments may be small enough to be dealt with by an individual or so large that there is a head of department, but in all cases there must be good liaison and communications are helped by a bleep system. (See page 282.)

Owing to the great variety of types of establishments it is not easy to give details of co-operation which would apply in all cases. For this reason a large hotel has been chosen as an example and the following are the departments with which there should be close co-operation.

Reception

Co-operation here is particularly necessary because the work of the two departments is very closely allied, and each must understand the other's difficulties. It is usual for hotels to state that rooms must be vacated by noon on the day of departure, but owing to the increased number of guests arriving early for one reason or another, new guests may arrive before the rooms have been serviced, and to avoid them being shown into untidy rooms, the housekeeper should notify the receptionists of 'ready rooms' as soon as they become available. She should also notify them when rooms are to be 'taken off' for redecoration, and again when they are 'put on'. At certain times of the day the housekeeper will let the receptionist have a control sheet (occupancy list, housekeeper's report or vacant room list) so that the receptionist may check the room-booking board or chart. The housekeeper relies on the receptionists to let her know arrivals and departures, when V.I.P.'s are expected, and when special requests have been made for cots, bed boards or baby sitters, etc. In large modern hotels tape recorders, tele-writers or room status boards may be installed to facilitate communications between the two departments.

Maintenance

In the course of the day the housekeeper finds many items requiring attention, such as dripping taps, W.C. cisterns not flushing, faulty electrical plugs or broken sash cords, and she should report these faults as early in the day as possible. If a good relationship exists between the two departments, notification of an urgent repair will be dealt with at once, and not just added to wait its turn on the list. However, it must be remembered that maintenance is required in other departments besides housekeeping, and thus co-operation is most important.

Restaurant

Co-operation here is mainly concerned with the linen, and while the linen keeper, under the supervision of the housekeeper, needs to have sufficient stock to meet the demands of the restaurant, the restaurant manager should ensure that the times for exchange of linen are respected, and that linen is not mis-used. However, with the greater use of plastics and disposable articles there is in some establishments very much less use of linen. Co-operation is particularly necessary where there is a floor waiter service, so that friction does not arise over such trivial matters as waiters not collecting trays from the rooms, or causing extra work through careless spills on carpets.

Kitchen

The same co-operation is necessary regarding linen as for the restaurant, and in addition, a happy atmosphere between the chef and the house-keeper, makes one important aspect of staff welfare, i.e. food, much less of a problem, as complaints may be discussed on a more friendly basis. The housekeeper can help by endeavouring to see that her staff are punctual for their meals and so avoid complaints from the kitchen.

Accounts

Wage packets are made up from the information received from the housekeeper regarding hours worked, holidays taken, days lost due to sickness, etc., and where this is accurate and punctual, it is hoped that the staff of the housekeeping department will not be kept waiting unnecessarily in a queue for their wage packets.

Head Porter

Co-operation with the head porter is necessary regarding lists for early morning teas and calls, the prompt removal of luggage from vacated rooms, and the willing loan of his staff when house porters are not available. The housekeeper and/or the linen keeper should co-operate by ensuring that the linen room key or a supply of linen is available for the night porter (when this is the house custom) in case of an emergency during the night.

Security

Co-operation here is mainly concerned with the prevention of fire and theft and the safe keeping of keys and lost property. There are so many security hazards on the 'floors' that liaison is particularly important and the housekeeper co-operates by endeavouring to see that her staff are aware of them.

Buyer

Co-operation is particularly important here so that there can be discussions between the two departmental heads over suitability versus costs of many items; it is desirable that the housekeeper should approve of a specific item before a large consignment is ordered and she should give due warning when she wants to change a certain type of article.

Laundry (where on premises under a Laundry Manager)

Without clean linen the maids cannot operate. At times when there is full occupancy the housekeeper needs a fast turn round of linen from the laundry but she should not always be making emergency demands on them. She should co-operate when possible with their normal scheduling and in return the laundry should provide an acceptable service in regard to the cleaning of the linen.

Recruitment and Training of Staff

Even when there is a personnel officer or staff manager, the *housekeeper* has the final decision regarding the selection of her staff. Where she is responsible for recruitment appointments should be made as quickly as possible, otherwise existing staff may become unco-operative at the extra work to be done. The following may be useful sources:

1 Advertisements in newspapers and trade journals—these should be as detailed as money allows and if a box number is used, the locality should be indicated. The most suitable papers and days may become known and advertisements should not be kept in too long or they may lose their effectiveness.
2 Private agencies—this may be an expensive method of recruitment as the agency normally demands a high fee from the employer.
3 Local Labour Employment Exchange and Youth Employment Service. It is useful to keep in contact with these people so that they know the *housekeeper's* particular requirements.
4 Cards in shop windows—this is a useful method of recruitment for local part-time labour.
5 Internal grape-vine—this may lead to the employment of friends and relatives of existing employees.
6 Former employees—the majority of workers leave voluntarily and over a period of time home ties and other circumstances change.
7 Colleges, schools, etc.—courses normally finish about the end of June, but there may be students available for evening, weekend or holiday jobs.

It may be useful to record the result of the methods employed for future reference and the following headings might be appropriate:

Source of Recruitment	Cost	Date	Response	Applicants employed

Where possible any suitable applicant should be called for interview and the following points are suggested for an inexperienced interviewer:

1 Full name and address—if the applicant is to be non-resident, this may lead to the pointing out of travel difficulties.
2 Age and place of birth—these should indicate whether the applicant is too near retiring age, too young for the rest of the staff, needs a work permit.
3 Qualifications and particulars of former jobs; reasons for changing.
4 Health and sick leave in the past—such things as shortness of breath, varicose veins, etc., may be noticed and lead to further questioning.
5 Family commitments—these are of importance where the applicant is to be non-resident and cover such points as husband's work, age of children.
6 Work and other relevant details discussed such as—hours, duties, wages, holidays, uniform, meal facilities, any deductions to be made from pay, e.g. sick scheme or superannuation, regulations concerning the searching of employees' bags as they leave the premises and if to be resident, the type of accommodation and where possible this should be shown, length of time for notice of leaving or dismissal (it is usual for a week's notice to be given on either side).
7 The applicant should be given an opportunity to ask questions.
8 Names and addresses and/or telephone number of referees.

During the interview the *housekeeper* will form certain impressions about the applicant, e.g. neatness, health, personal hygiene, politeness, cheerful or moody disposition and from this knowledge the *housekeeper* should be better able to decide where and with whom the applicant could work and live.

After the *housekeeper* has summed up the suitability of the applicant for the work and having asked for the name, address and telephone number of a former employer and/or another referee she will take up references. As many employers are often unwilling to commit themselves on paper, particularly in the case of doubtful employees, it is not unusual to obtain a verbal reference by telephone. However, this would not provide a permanent record, so the referee should be asked to follow up the conversation with a letter which can then be filed. If the references are taken up by telephone towards the end of the interview, it may be possible to engage the applicant straight away. She should be told the date she is to begin work and asked to bring from her last employer the form (P45) showing the amount she has earned and the income tax paid, as well as her National Insurance Card. It is advisable for a *housekeeper* to have a knowledge of the legal aspects regarding such things as the employment of foreign labour, National Insurance, Graduated Pensions, contracts of employment and Union requirements.

Once the applicant is engaged, training becomes necessary. Good induction at the commencement of their employment enables the new employees to settle in more quickly; it is hoped that during this period they are made to feel that they belong and are a necessary part of the establishment. They may be shown the whereabouts of the canteen, cloakrooms, linen room, various offices, stores, etc., and briefed regarding the necessity of personal hygiene, courtesy, security, safety and fire precautions and the need to ask if instructions are not clear. During this period many points raised at the interview—e.g. conditions of service, pay, holidays, etc.—may be explained more fully.

Following this introduction, if the induction period is sufficiently long the maids may be given some 'off the job' training in technical skills by a trained instructor when full use should be made of cleaning equipment, agents and methods for the different jobs.

There is an old saying

> I hear —I forget
> I see   —I remember
> I do   —I understand

To this end, in any 'off the job' training, talks should be kept short, demonstrations given and ample time allowed for employees to try out equipment, use agents, etc., and ask questions.

Whether there has been any training in technical skills during the induction period or not, once the maid is 'on the job' training will still be necessary. This may be carried out by 'working with Nellie' but this is hardly an adequate method unless Nellie is a willing and carefully selected worker who might be given an incentive bonus. An alternative method would be by the use of 'order of work' cards or training manual under the direct supervision of an assistant housekeeper—or better still would be 'on the job' training by a trained member of staff.

Further 'off the job' training should be included in the training programme and may involve lectures, demonstrations and audience participation.

In some spheres the H.C.I.T.B. is trying to improve training and redistribute money for this purpose throughout the country. Its objectives as outlined by the Industrial Training Act are: to ensure an adequate supply of properly trained men and women at all levels in industry; to secure an improvement in the quality and efficiency of industrial training; to share the cost of training more evenly between employers. Housekeepers and their assistants may have the opportunity of attending the H.C.I.T.B. Instructors' Training Courses or refresher courses which might be arranged at technical colleges. Where assistant housekeepers are quite inexperienced they may attend block release or short courses.

The National Health Service is out of the scope of the Industrial Training Act and the Department of Health and Social Security has the Advisory Committee on Ancillary Staff Training to provide guidelines to the Health Service on the training of Ancillary Staff Grades, e.g. domestic, catering, portering and laundry staff, etc.

Welfare of staff

Good employees are difficult to get, and once obtained it is up to the *housekeeper* to be concerned with their welfare in order that they will stay.

Residential establishments have to compete with factories and offices where staff work a 5-day week, while the housekeeping staff in some places have to man the department 14–16 hours a day for 7 days a week. This is often a bone of contention with staff and in order to make the hours more acceptable to them, the *housekeeper* tries to arrange straight shifts rather than split duties. Due consideration should be given to wages, holidays and distribution of hours on duty. Maids should be compensated in some way for extra work done, as for example when there are no relief maids for days off, sickness or holidays. Incentive bonuses may be a means of motivating staff. Consideration might be given to moving maids round so that they do not always carry out the same work, and also to the possibility of maids working together on a job.

The Catering Wages Order, the Whitley Council and other bodies lay down minimum wages and holidays, and maximum working hours per week for different types of establishments and different grades of workers, and these regulations must be complied with when planning duty rosters and holiday lists. The planning of holiday lists can be a real problem as a minimum number of staff is required at any one time, but maids may have husbands at work, children at school and friends with whom they wish to spend their holidays, so holiday arrangements should be made early with as much consideration given to the individual as possible.

The feeding of her staff is not really the province of the *housekeeper* but in the interests of their welfare she is concerned that they have sufficient time to cover the distance between working areas and staff canteen, possibly to queue for and to eat their meals. Once there, there should be sufficient seating accommodation, clean table, cutlery and china for them to enjoy adequate and varied meals of the correct temperature and if there are complaints, the *housekeeper* should deal with them.

In the past maids had to accept cold, bare attics and basements as their 'homes' but today living-in staff need comfort and warmth, single rooms if possible, as well as a lockable cupboard, facilities for laundry and for making a hot drink, to encourage them to stay. For security reasons it is necessary to have individual lockers in which non-resident staff may keep their overalls, outdoor clothes and handbags.

Unless a *housekeeper* recognises each maid as an individual and not just as another pair of hands there may be instability and discontentment amongst the staff. This may give rise to resentment showing itself in the breaking of rules, absenteeism or stirring up trouble. In order that maids are made to feel that they and their work are important the *housekeeper* should show an interest, check a few rooms herself and give an occasional word of praise. In this way a happier atmosphere is created and less ill-feeling results when it is necessary to find fault. Any fault-finding should be done in private. In addition to knowing the names of her staff, the *housekeeper* should know something of their lives apart from their work and this knowledge will enable her to understand, sympathise and make allowances in individual performance.

A wise *housekeeper* will not make more rules for her staff than is absolutely necessary, but those that she makes, for example, no cardigans over uniforms, no jewellery, no smoking when on duty, must be enforced.

A maid in an hotel is usually allowed to turn the radio on low in the room in which she is working and normally she works with the door open. This, however, does present problems because the maid may be taken unawares by the guest or an intruder entering the room, particularly if the vacuum cleaner is working. The housekeeper should endeavour to see that her maids realise the need for safety, not only for the guest, for the guests' and hotel's property but also for themselves. There are hotels where the maids do not take early morning tea into rooms let to a man on his own, in order to overcome the possibility of advances by the opposite sex.

The *housekeeper* must have strict key control and her staff must understand the need for the correct use of keys. Loss of a master key may lead to dismissal (see p. 236).

Dissatisfaction may arise from the word 'chamber' maid, which originates from the French chambre meaning room, but to many people and students in particular, the word has other associations, and thus it might seem sensible to find a more pleasing name, e.g. room-maid.

It is usual for there to be some uniformity of dress for maids and in some establishments for assistant housekeepers also, and when it is possible to make changes the *housekeeper* should give careful consideration to the material, style and colour, so that the choice is not only comfortable for work but pleasing to the majority of the wearers. Since she may be asked to advise on the choice of uniform, furnishings and decoration, it would be wise for her to keep up-to-date with modern developments.

There is an increasing tendency for establishments, especially hotels, to have fewer staff living on the premises, so assistant housekeepers and maids may live in the establishment, live out or live in a house or hostel belonging to the establishment, when transport may be provided. The hours of duty will vary tremendously from one establishment to another (see Chapter 2) and these may be 38–44 hours with 1½–2 days off a week; some split duties may still be necessary, when a sitting-room should be available for non-resident staff.

Some maids make reliable assistant housekeepers but it is better that promotion is not within the same establishment, and for the new assistant housekeeper's own good it might be suggested that she does not tell her colleagues that she was previously working as a room-maid. The aim of an assistant is to become a *housekeeper* and while she is an assistant in an hotel, her wages are probably little, if any, more than the maids (who may work overtime and may get tips), but status is given to her in that, if resident, she has a single bedroom, takes her meals in the stewards' room (in newer hotels there may be a canteen where all staff feed) and she may or may not wear a uniform, according to house custom.

An enterprising *housekeeper* will not only train a deputy, but she will encourage her assistants to widen their knowledge, informing them of available lectures and classes on such things as a foreign language, First Aid and floral arrangement and making the necessary adjustments in their timetables so that they may attend.

It is usual for there to be a housekeeper's office where the *housekeeper* may discuss the affairs of the day with her assistants and where they may sit and do necessary paper work such as maintenance reports, rosters, records, etc.

The *housekeeper* should not get so immersed in paper work that she stays in her office all day; she should be seen about the house observing people and things, in other words having 'time to stand and stare' and in order to be contacted she should carry a 'bleep' (see p. 282). To gain this time, she has to delegate work to her assistants such as:

The keeping of record books.
The maids' rosters and holiday lists.
The training of the maids on the job.
The supervision of the stores and linen room.

The despatch and receipt of the dry cleaning articles.
The floral arrangements.

However, it must be emphasised that delegation does not mean the loss of responsibility, but the entrusting of it to a deputy.

In supervising and controlling her staff on duty, the *housekeeper* is concerned with their personal hygiene and appearance. Thus the *house-keeper* needs to train her maids in personal hygiene, in particular making them realise the importance of the cleanliness of all parts of the body, e.g. hands, nails, feet and hair, and the necessity for suitable clean clothing, including shoes and stockings when on duty. She herself should at all times be an example that they can look up to and respect. Employees tend either to look up to or down on their superiors, and the *housekeeper's* attitude sets the tone of the whole department. The staff take their cue from her so she should at all times be an example that they can look up to and respect. Courtesy and good manners are essential and in the hotel all guests should be addressed as 'Sir' or 'Madam'.

A *housekeeper* needs to provide up-to-date equipment and methods of work to save the time and energy of the staff. She needs to be a good disciplinarian and be firm regarding the rules that she makes. In order to keep her staff she must realise there will be times when she has to give way and in doing so she must be just and fair and avoid favouritism.

A good *housekeeper* will always have the welfare of her staff at heart and be prepared to stand up for them at all times.

The status of the *housekeeper* varies considerably depending on her experience, length of service, strength of character and personality as well as on the size of the establishment and whether it is in the commercial or welfare field. Depending on her status, her accommodation may be a self-contained flat, a suite or a bed-sitting room, or she may be non-resident.

A housekeeper's attributes should include:

An interest in people and tact in handling them.
A pleasant personality and the ability to converse with all types of people.
An ability to hide personal likes and dislikes, and to be conscientious, fair and just.
Strictness regarding punctuality and the keeping of necessary rules.
Loyalty to the hotel and to her staff.
Critical powers of observation.
A sense of humour.
An adaptability and willingness to experiment with new ideas, use initiative and take responsibility.

A cool head to deal with any emergencies.

The possession of a strong heart and good feet.

For all these attributes to be incorporated in one person would make her a paragon and such a person rarely exists, thus a few of these can be missing if a *housekeeper* has a sense of humour and a pleasing personality.

To sum up, it may be said that while a *housekeeper*'s life is a busy one, requiring patience, skill and good humour, it is also a very varied and satisfying one.

In the past the field of housekeeping was almost entirely confined to women but now, with the wider concept of housekeeping, men are becoming more involved and there is a greater need for them to study the rudiments of housekeeping.

2

The Organisation of the Housekeeping Department

As the housekeeping department plays such a large part in the economic running of an establishment, a good *housekeeper* should, while maintaining efficiency throughout the department, save as much on operating costs as possible. Methods which she may employ to achieve this end include work study, the forecasting of labour requirements in relation to room occupancy, and budgeting and these are dealt with more fully in Chapter 16.

The organisation of the housekeeping department is therefore a very real job, and without good organisation there may be repercussions throughout the house.

In order that her staff may work efficiently, the *housekeeper* should see that they have suitable equipment, have suitable cleaning materials and use the best methods.

Equipment

Cleaning is the removal of dust, dirt and any foreign matter, e.g. dead flowers, stains, contents of ashtrays and waste-paper baskets, etc., and it is necessary for hygienic reasons, for the sake of appearance and to prevent deterioration.

Removal of dust

Dust is loose particles which are frequently airborne, and later settle on any surface, and it is essential that during the removal of dust the particles are collected and not merely shifted from one place to another.

The removal of dust is an important part of the work of the housekeeping staff, and its collection may be by sweeping, mopping, dusting or suction.

After it has been collected, dust may be disposed of by burning, putting down a rubbish chute, emptying into a paper sack or dustbin which will later be emptied by a houseporter (if the dust is first wrapped in paper, the emptying and cleaning of the bin is much easier and far more hygienic) or, if collected on a mop or duster, by shaking and occasionally washing.

When removing dust from a variety of surfaces in a room, it may be necessary to use several methods for its removal, e.g. sweeping, dusting, mopping and vacuum cleaning, and these should be used in that order.

Thus, where several methods are to be used, a room having a polished surround to a carpet square may be cleaned in the following order:

1 Dust all surfaces.

2 Mop surround.

3 Vacuum clean upholstery and carpet.

or

1 Sweep upholstery and surround.

2 Dust all surfaces.

3 Vacuum clean carpet.

Brooms and brushes are used for the removal of dust from a variety of surfaces, floors, walls, upholstery, clothes, etc., and may have bristles of animal, vegetable or man-made origin.

Most brooms and brushes have a stock of wood or plastic into which bristles are fixed. Handles join the stock, and these are now frequently painted or made of plastic, and are therefore less likely to splinter and are more easily cleaned with a damp cloth, than the older plain wooden handles.

In order to keep the bristles in good condition, brooms and brushes must never rest on their bristles; when not in use brooms should be hung up on hooks or holders. They must be kept clean and after use any fluff, bits of

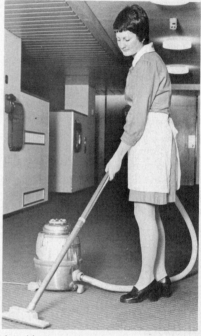

A maid vacuum cleaning

cotton or hair should be removed, and when necessary the brushes should be washed in warm water and detergent, rinsed, shaken free of surplus water, and left to dry so that the water does not seep into the wooden stock. Stiff bristles should be finally rinsed in cold, salt water to keep them stiff. Nylon bristles wash and dry easily, but are inclined to be springy and so disperse the dust when being used.

In the past a soft broom was used on hard floors and a stiff one on carpets, however, sweeping raises a certain amount of dust and, with the advent of the more hygienic process of vacuum cleaning, the use of the broom is becoming less and less. Brooms and brushes should not be used in hospitals as it is important that dust does not become airborne and spread infection.

Cobwebs may be removed as well as dust from cornices, picture rails and high ledges by the use of a broom with a long handle which is usually made of cane for lightness. The head may be of soft hair or feathers.

Dusting mops are used for the collection of dust from a polished floor and consist of a head made from soft twisted cotton yarn or synthetic fibres attached to a handle; the synthetic fibres are electrostatic and hold the dust more easily. The loose dust particles are removed by shaking and when dirty the mophead should be washed. Some cotton mopheads are impregnated with oil when they are known as mop sweepers and the dust then adheres more satisfactorily. When dirty, the head should be washed, dried and re-impregnated and the provision of clean mopheads may be a contract service.

Dusters are used for the collection of dust from hard surfaces and are usually made of soft cotton or short-life material. Dusting is only an effective method of the removal of dust when the dust is actually collected on the duster. This entails the duster being used in the form of a pad with no loose ends to flick the dust about. Damp dusting (using a swab, mutton cloth or short-life cloth) may prove more effective on some surfaces and is the only method used in hospitals. Dusters should be washed frequently. N.B. The yellow ones have a very loose dye.

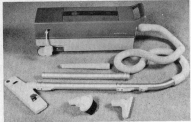 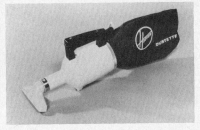

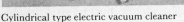

Cylindrical type electric vacuum cleaner   Dustette

A carpet or box sweeper is used for the removal of loose particles from carpets (some can be used on other floorings). It consists of a revolving brush between two small dustpans, on four rubber covered wheels, motivated by the worker, and requires frequent emptying. Fluff and bits of cotton should be removed from the bristles and round the wheels, and occasionally the brush should be washed, and the moving parts oiled for ease of movement, and to prevent squeaking.

Electric vacuum cleaners are used for the removal of dust by suction from any surface, hard or soft. The dust is collected into a container, which may be enclosed within the body of the machine, or on the

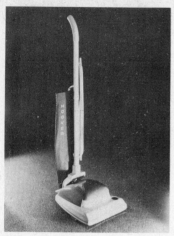

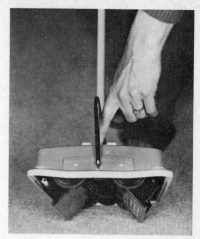

Upright electric vacuum cleaner   Manually operated carpet sweeper

outside in the form of a bag. Some are more adaptable for special purposes than others, and the choice will therefore rest on the main work that is to be done with the machine.

It is essential that the bag or container into which the dust collects is not allowed to become overfull, or a strain is put on the motor. Damage to the cotton bag should be avoided and it should never be washed or it will allow dust as well as air to pass through it.

With all electrical equipment regular servicing is necessary; flex and plug defects, and unusual working noises should be reported immediately; unqualified persons should not try their hand at repairs. When machines break down (and they often do, owing to careless use), repairs may take some time and during this period the lack of equipment may present difficulties, so some establishments have their electrical equipment, e.g. vacuum cleaners, polishers, etc., on hire, the firms being under contract to supply the required number of items in working order.

It is possible to have a centralised vacuum cleaning system built into an establishment, where ducts carry dust direct to a basement dust room and the spread of micro-organisms is avoided. (Micro-organisms may be carried through the bag of the mobile vacuum cleaner even when a diaphragm filter is fitted.) There are outlets from the ducts into which the cleaning operators insert a hose to which they attach a suitable nozzle for the particular job. This system is better built into a new building, as afterwards it is expensive to install; the storage of hoses may be a problem and unless lightweight hose is used, it is heavy for women to operate, but there are no frayed flexes and no individual machines to go wrong or to be emptied.

Removal of dirt

Dirt is dust or other material which, by means of grease or moisture, adheres to a surface, and its removal may be by the use of a grease solvent and/or by washing, mopping, shampooing or scrubbing, when friction must be applied in conjunction with hot water, a detergent and possibly an abrasive. The loosened dirt and water are removed by means of a cloth, a mop or a vacuum drying machine.

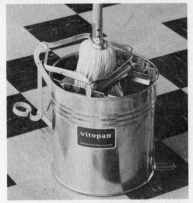

Vitopan mini mop

Brushes are used for the removal of dirt from a variety of surfaces such as floors, W.C. pans, upholstery, etc. Scrubbing by hand, using a scrubbing brush in conjunction with a floor cloth, detergent and warm water was the accepted method for the removal of dirt from hard floors, but now large areas are cleaned by a scrubbing brush on a long handle (deck scrubber) or scrubbing machines in conjunction with a mop or a vacuum drying machine.

Scrubbing machines consist of one large or several small brushes which revolve and scrub the floor; the water and detergent are released from a tank attached to the machine. With suitable brushes these machines can be used for shampooing carpets, polishing, spray buffing or spray cleaning floors.

A wet mop or a sponge mop is used for cleaning lightly soiled floors in conjunction with a bucket, water and detergent; for large areas the bucket may be on castors and have a wringer attachment. The mop consists of longer, coarser cotton yarn than a dry mop and a sponge mop is another type of wet mop. Both these mops, unless washed well after use, become unhygienic.

Cloths. A variety of cloths is needed for cleaning and protection, and they must be kept clean. The following four cloths are normally used for wet work, and each of them must be absorbent and of a manageable size, to enable them to be wrung out by hand.

Swabs may be of mutton cloth or other soft, absorbent material and are usually about 45 cm square. They are used for wet work above the floor, i.e. washing paint, baths, lavatory basins, etc., and they should be washed, opened out and allowed to dry after use to prevent them from becoming unhygienic.

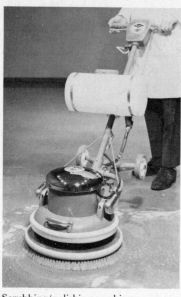 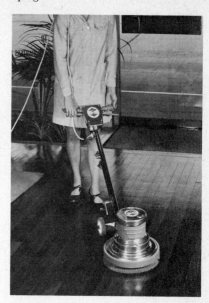

Scrubbing/polishing machines

Floor cloths are made of coarser cotton material than swabs, and are used for floors and W.C. pedestals. They should be washed and dried after use. It is wise to use a kneeling mat when cleaning a floor by hand.

Chamois leathers were originally the skins of the chamois goats, but now they are usually skivers, i.e. split skins of the sheep. They are used wet for cleaning windows and mirrors, but they are also used dry as a polishing cloth for silver. They should be washed when necessary, and rubbed when dry to soften them. As they are expensive they are only issued as required for special jobs.

Scrim is a loosely woven linen material, and because of its absorbency and not leaving linters, it is often used instead of chamois leather for cleaning windows and mirrors.

For dry work dusters and rags are used.

Dusters are of two types, checked cotton material and yellow flannelette; the latter is perhaps softer and better for highly polished surfaces, but has a very loose dye. They must be washed frequently and their approximate size is 50 cm square. Nowadays disposable dusters may be used.

Rag may be obtained from the linen room or bought by the sack and is used for applying polish, and when it is dirty it is thrown away.

The following cloths are used to protect surfaces:

Dust sheets are made of thin cotton material, and may be 'discards' from the linen room, e.g. thin curtains and bedspreads. When bought they are usually about the size of a single sheet. They must always be kept clean and are used for covering furniture, stored articles, and during spring cleaning.

Hearth cloths are made of hessian or American cloth, and their size varies. They are used to protect the carpet and floor when a fireplace is being cleaned, and they must be kept clean. They are rarely used now as coal fires have been replaced by central heating.

Bucket cloths or Splash mats may be as above, but much smaller. They are used by window cleaners and anyone using a bucket, to prevent marking a carpet or polished floor.

Druggets are made of coarse linen or fine canvas, and may be in the form of a 'carpet square' or a runner. They are used to protect the floor during bad weather and during redecoration.

Containers. A variety of containers is useful when cleaning and their condition is the responsiblity of the user.

Housemaids' or Chambermaids' boxes were originally made of wood or metal but nowadays are made of plastic. They consist of a box with a handle and a fitted tray, and are used by maids for carrying small items, e.g. toilet soap, polishes, abrasives, cloths, etc., and a plastic bucket is a fair substitute.

Trolleys may be used when a maid's section is all on one level, the corridor wide enough and there is sufficient storage space. A trolley is a large fitted conveyance, which as well as holding the items mentioned for the housemaid's box, has a bag for soiled linen and one for rubbish, shelves on which clean linen and other accessories are carried and also a step on which the vacuum cleaner rests.

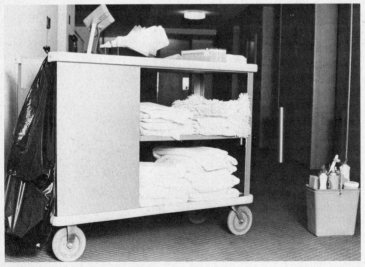

A chambermaid's box and trolley

Buckets (pails) are normally made of plastic these days because they are lighter in weight, much quieter in use, and very much easier to clean than galvanised iron ones. A mop bucket is still made of galvanised iron, in order that it can withstand the strain imposed when a mop is twisted or wrung in it.

Dustpans are used in conjunction with a brush for the gathering of dust. Formerly they were of metal but now plastic ones are more usual and in order to be effective, the edge in contact with the floor must be thin and flat.

Dustbins are often kept on the back stairs or in the maids' service room. They used to be of galvanised iron and were very noisy, but now they may be of rubber composition or they may be in the form of refuse sacks, which are strong disposable paper sacks attached to a stand.

Sanibins are small metal or plastic containers with lids, found in toilets for the collection of soiled sanitary towels. The bins must be emptied frequently and kept clean and for hygienic reasons paper bags are often provided for the wrapping of the soiled towels. In some places, incinerators have been installed to replace sanibins and these burn the towels leaving a small amount of ash which has to be removed during cleaning, or alternatively a 'Personnel Hygiene Service' may be in use when the container is on loan and changed regularly (see page 230).

Choice of equipment

When choosing equipment it is important that the right piece is chosen for the job and is suitable for the user. The cost and the efficiency of the piece of equipment and the time and labour saved by the user must all be taken into consideration.

It may be wise to have the article on a trial period when it can be decided whether it is

of good quality;
easy to empty and clean;
easy to get replacements;
noisy;
too heavy for the user;
too cumbersome;
safe in operation;
easy to use and not too complicated.

Often a large expensive piece of equipment cannot be fully utilised and to help overcome this waste a dual-purpose machine might be considered.

Having decided on the type of article the final purchase will depend on the

servicing arrangements;
length of guarantee;
price.

Care of equipment

Having selected and bought good equipment it is up to the *housekeeper* to see that it is properly looked after. This means that training and good supervision are necessary and she should ensure that the staff

use it properly;
store it correctly;
are given time to clean it;
realise the importance of reporting faults promptly.

Cleaning Agents

Dust, being loose particles, is comparatively easily removed by the use of various pieces of equipment; dirt, however, owing to its adhering to surfaces by means of grease or moisture, requires the use of cleaning agents as well as equipment, if it is to be removed efficiently.

Water is the simplest cleaning agent, and some forms of dirt will be dissolved by it, but normally unless it is used in conjunction with some other agent, for example a detergent, water is not an effective cleanser. In fact it does not even wet a surface satisfactorily as its surface tension prevents it from spreading.

Detergents are cleaning agents which when used in conjunction with water can loosen and remove dirt, and then hold it in suspension so that the dirt is not redeposited on the clean surface.

There is a large number of detergents available and in general, powdered ones are designed for the washing of fabrics and liquid ones for washing up and the cleaning of hard surfaces such as floors, etc. They all consist of complex mixtures of chemical substances and while the term is frequently applied to synthetic soapless detergents only, it does strictly include soaps. Detergents may therefore be in cake, powder or liquid form and the basic ingredients are surfactants (surface active agents). These are the wetting agents which lower the surface tension of the water and to varying degrees emulsify and suspend greasy dirt.

Detergency is brought about by the molecules of the surfactant having one end which is attracted to water (hydrophilic) and the other which is repelled by water (hydrophobic) and is attracted to grease. Because of the nature of the molecules the grease and dirt is lifted from the surface and held in suspension.

It is the hydrophobic part of the molecule which activates the cleaning process. When dissolved in water, some surfactants ionise or split up into positively and negatively charged particles called ions while others do not and surfactants are classified on this basis.

Anionic surfactants are those which carry a negative charge on the larger ion or active constituent.

Cationic surfactants carry a positive charge on the larger ion.

Non-ionic surfactants do not ionise in solution but they still have the hydrophobic/hydrophilic nature.

All soaps are anionic, e.g. sodium stearate ionising into the large and active ion with its negative charge and the smaller metal ion with its positive charge.

$$C_{17}H_{35}COO\ Na \rightleftharpoons C_{17}H_{35}COO^- + Na^+$$

Any anionic surfactant can be mixed with other anionics or with non-ionics but they cannot be combined with cationics.

The anionics constitute the largest group of surfactants and are used extensively in powdered detergents. However powdered detergents do normally consist of a mixture of anionic and non-ionic surfactants with the latter incorporated in comparatively small amounts to modify the amount of lather formed by the powdered product.

In a liquid product non-ionics are used because of their high solubility. (Cationic cannot be mixed with anionic ones and their use in detergents is therefore limited but they do have good germicidal properties. 'Quats' or quaternary ammonium compounds are probably the most important of the cationics.)

An important consideration in choosing surfactants for a detergent base is that they should be biodegradable, that is, they should break down in rivers and sewage works waters.

To formulate a successful detergent several other ingredients are normally added to the mixture of surfactants; these additives aid the emulsifying and suspending powers of the detergent and their nature and amounts will depend on the purpose for which the particular detergent is intended. In general, powdered detergents will contain more additives than liquid ones as the former are intended to be heavy duty detergents used for the washing of soiled fabrics. Some of the more frequently added substances are:

Inorganic builders which are alkaline salts such as soda, borates, silicates or complex phosphates, and these increase the efficiency of cleansing by assisting in the softening of the water and enabling more of the surfactant to remove the dirt. The complex phosphates are sequestering agents and block the calcium and magnesium of the hard water forming no scum. The major role of sodium silicate is to prevent the corrosion of metals especially aluminium and act as a preservative (an anti-oxidant) for soap. Mixtures of alkaline builders and surfactants often give greater efficiency than would be expected when considering the efficiency of the individual components. The mixtures are then said to be synergistic. The addition of these alkaline salts obviously increases the alkalinity of the detergent powder and this will result in most cases, of a pH about 9. Powdered detergents may contain as much as 30% inorganic builders. These detergents with a high pH value should not be used for the washing of the skin nor of animal fibres (wool, silk) which are sensitive to high alkalinity.

Sodium Carboxy Methyl Cellulose (SCMC) which assists the suspending power of the detergent and thus helps prevent dirt re-settling on the clean article.

Sodium perborate which is an oxidising bleach added to remove stains of tea, coffee, fruit juice, etc., but is only effective at high temperatures (most effective above 80°C) or after long soaking at lower temperatures.

Foam boosters or stabilisers which increase and stabilise the suds so that the suds serve as an indicator of the amount of detergent power left in the solution.

Brightening agents which absorb ultra violet light and convert it to visible light thus making the fabric appear brighter.

Enzymes which enable the removal of protein stains such as blood, egg and perspiration. They are biological catalysts and work most effectively around temperatures of 40-50°C or during prolonged soaks at lower temperatures.

Germicides, perfumes and dye stuffs may be added. Perfumes are used to give a clean fresh fragrance and only in toilet soap to give a scent in the normal meaning.

Detergents may, therefore, contain many ingredients and this is particularly true of the powdered ones, both soap and synthetic, and according to the composition of the mixture, each detergent will have advantages for a particular cleaning job.

In order that the washing process should be carried out efficiently, an ideal detergent should

have good wetting powers so that the solution penetrates between the article and the dirt particles;

have good emulsifying powers so that grease and oil are broken up and to some extent dissolved;

have good suspending powers so that the dirt particles, when

removed, are suspended in the solution and are not redeposited on
the article;

be readily soluble in water;

be effective in all types of water and produce no scum;

be effective over a wide range of temperatures;

be harmless to the article and the skin;

cleanse reasonably quickly and with minimum agitation.

Soap is obtained when fat or oil is treated with an alkali (saponification), and is an anionic surfactant.

When used for cleaning, soap is cheap and effective in soft water, but in hard water it does not lather readily and it forms a scum which is difficult to rinse away. In order to overcome this, alkaline 'builders' generally in the form of soda or complex phosphates, are added to household soaps; these assist in the removal of the hardness of the water and in breaking up the grease and oil.

Although soap has in many instances been superseded by the synthetic (soapless) detergents, cakes of toilet soap still remain.

Toilet soap. The work toilet soap has to do is not particularly heavy, and since the cleansing is done by means of a lather which has a fairly high concentration of soap, there is no need for builders. Hence toilet soaps are generally unbuilt; they do, however, contain perfumes, dyestuffs and possibly anti-oxidants.

In hotels gross boxes of 22 g and 56 g tablets are usual, and these may be wrapped with the name of the hotel printed on the soap or the wrapping, or unwrapped when careful storage is necessary, in order that the soap retains its fresh appearance. The tablets are issued for use in the guests' rooms, private bathrooms, and cloakrooms, and pieces left over from the guests' rooms may be transferred to the cloakrooms for general use, or returned to the manufacturer for remaking, when a slight discount is given.

Scrubbing soap contains builders and about 30 per cent. water, and is generally bought in bars of 453 g.

Soap flakes, because of their immense surface area compared with the same weight of soap, dissolve more easily and yield quicker suds. They are expensive and are generally unbuilt and may be used for the laundering of delicate fabrics. They may be bought in packets or in bulk.

Soap powders dissolve and lather faster than bar soap, because of the great surface area for a given weight of soap. They often contain large quantities of builders, some as much as 40 per cent. and so can be formulated to cleanse more efficiently than bar soap. They may be bought in packets or in bulk.

Synthetic (soapless) detergents have replaced the use of soap in many cleaning processes because they are not affected by hard water, have good suspending powers, do not dry smeary and most are stable in acidic or alkaline media, (however soap is not effective in acid solution). It is for these reasons that as long as the water containing the synthetic detergent remains clean, there is no need to rinse hard surfaces such as walls, floors, etc.

Liquid synthetic (soapless) detergents are basically solutions of the surfactants with the necessary additional substances added, and processed in such a way that the various ingredients do not separate with temperature changes. Due to fewer builders being added these liquid detergents are nearer neutral in reaction and may have a pH7. They are satisfactory for the cleaning of hard surfaces, and washing up, but are not satisfactory for heavily soiled fabrics and have no great suspending powers. They are reasonably economical in use, and are effective with a minimum of lather.

Powdered synthetic detergents are manufactured to a far greater extent than the liquid ones. Every type contains many ingredients, i.e. builders and other necessary substances, and by altering the proportions, the particular detergent may become more suitable for one purpose than another.

Synthetic detergents will be used for a great variety of purposes including washing up, and the washing of floors, walls, baths, basins and fabrics and may be bought in bulk or in smaller containers.

Biological detergents contain enzymes.

Abrasives depend on their rubbing or scratching action to clean dirt from hard surfaces. The extent to which they will rub or scratch a surface, depends on the nature of the abrasive material, and the size and shape of the particles.

Glass, sand and emery papers are all forms of abrasives, as are steel wool, nylon web pads, powdered pumice, fine ash, precipitated whiting (filtered chalk) and jewellers' rouge (a pink oxide of iron), the last two being the finest. The use of abrasives will depend on the surface to be cleaned and the type of dirt to be removed and when possible fine abrasives should be used in preference to coarser ones.

Scouring powders are made from fine particles of pumice mixed with soap or a synthetic detergent, an alkali to remove grease, and often a small quantity of chlorine bleach. Their exact composition will vary with the brand and whereas they were originally made with a view to cleaning baths and lavatory basins they now have a much wider use, e.g. the removal of rubber heel marks from hard floors. Although they are fine abrasives they will scratch surfaces if used too generously. They should be applied on a damp cloth and well rinsed away.

Scouring pastes are normally milder in their action than scouring powders. The fine abrasive powder is mixed with soap to which a small amount of alkali is added, and often some glycerine. The pastes are used in the same way as the powders and are probably more economical, as they are not spilt or tipped over so easily, but they do become dried up if stored for too long.

Scouring liquids are still milder in their abrasive action. They generally contain ammonia to aid the removal of grease and need to be well shaken before use so that the abrasive powder is not left at the bottom of the container.

Toilet Cleansers are crystalline or liquid and they rely on their acid content to clean and keep the W.C. pan hygienic. The crystalline ones are normally based on sodium acid sulphate, a mild acid which is mixed with an anti-caking agent, often pine oil which also helps prevent corrosion of any metal container. The cleansing effect can be improved by the addition of a small amount of acid resistant anionic surfactant. The liquid cleansers may contain hydrochloric acid and should only be used as directed.

Toilet cleansers should never under any circumstances be used for anything other than W.C. pans, nor should they ever be mixed with any other cleansers or harmful gases are likely to be produced.

Window cleansers consist of a water miscible solvent, often isopropyl alcohol, to which a small quantity of synthetic detergent and possibly an alkali, are added to improve the polishing effect of the cleanser. Some also contain a fine abrasive. The cleanser is applied with a cleaning rag and rubbed off with a clean, soft cloth.

Water, or water to which some methylated spirit has been added, does the job quite well and much more cheaply but entails more rubbing.

Soda and ammonia are alkalis, and are used as grease emulsifiers and stain removal agents. The addition of alkaline salts to surfactants in the formulation of detergents has already been mentioned.

Strong alkaline cleaning agents based on caustic soda in flake or liquid form are available for the cleaning of blocked drains, cleaning ovens and other large industrial equipment. Extreme care has to be taken in their use as they are very strong materials with high pH values. (1% solution may have a pH of 13.1.)

Vinegar and lemon (cut or juice) are acids, and are used for the removal of mild water stains on baths, etc. More resistant stains may be removed with stronger acids such as **oxalic acid** or **spirits of salt** (concentrated hydrochloric acid). These should only be used under strict supervision, and in all cases of cleaning the acids must be thoroughly rinsed away or they may harm the surface.

(There is a variety of proprietary substances sold under trade names which are helpful in the removal of hard water deposits.)

Paraffin oil is also efficient for the cleaning of baths but owing to its smell is seldom used.

Methylated spirit, white spirit (turpentine substitute) and **carbon tetrachloride** are grease solvents, and used for the removal of grease and wax from different surfaces. The two former are highly inflammable while carbon tetrachloride is harmful if inhaled, and should therefore never be used in a confined space.

Aerosol dry cleansers suitable for use on wallpaper and furnishings are available.

Bleaches used for cleaning purposes are generally alkaline stabilised solutions of sodium hypochlorite, and are useful for stained sinks, W.C. pans, etc. but they should never be mixed with other types of toilet cleansers. They whiten and have germicidal properties and great care should be taken to prevent spotting of other surfaces. Other bleaches are mentioned in connection with the removal of stains from fabrics on p. 97.

Disinfectants, antiseptics and **deodorants** are not strictly cleaning agents, but are often used during cleaning operations. The use of disinfectants and antiseptics should be controlled carefully, as many have strong smells and their use often suggests illness or bad drains.

Disinfectants kill bacteria; antiseptics prevent bacterial growth and are frequently diluted disinfectants; deodorants mask unpleasant smells either by combining chemically with the particles forming the smell, or by their smell being predominant. All of these may be obtained as aerosol sprays.

Quaternary ammonium compounds (cationic surfactants) are useful bacteriocides and deodorants but they cannot be used with anionic soaps or soapless detergents.

Polishes provide a shine, and some clean at the same time, while many provide a protective coating to the surface. They may be used on floors, walls, furniture, leather or metals and their composition will depend on the surface for which they are intended. There are new brands of polishes coming on the market continually and in general the requirements of a good polish are that:

it is non greasy;
it gives a good shine easily;
it does not mark;
it does not smell unpleasant;
it should give a hard dry finish to ensure maximum protection and ease of cleaning.

The glossy appearance of a polished surface is due to the reflection of light from the smooth surface. Originally it was thought that friction or buffing was necessary to produce the smooth surface but new developments have shown that this is not always the case and that smooth surfaces can be produced by

(a) a layer of material from the polish itself, e.g. a wax film left on floors or furniture after the spirit solvent and/or water present evaporates. The gloss may or may not be intensified by buffing.

(b) a layer of the polished material itself smoothed by the frictional heat generated during polishing e.g. metals, when the cleaning action of the abrasives and other substances gives the shiny surface.

Floor polishes consist of blends of natural waxes and synthetic resins and are of two main types:

1　Spirit based floor waxes or polishes
2　Water based floor waxes or polishes

1　*Spirit based floor polishes* are blends of mainly natural waxes dispersed in a spirit solvent, originally turpentine but now more often white spirit. The amount of spirit added determines the consistency of the polish which may be paste or liquid. The additional solvent in the liquid polish increases the cleaning action of the polish, although it should still only be applied to a dust free floor.

Some of the paste polishes contain silicones. These are complex substances containing silicon and because of their low surface tension they make the wax easier to apply. They have water repellent properties and help in the formation of a hard, glossy film but they tend to increase slipperiness and are therefore more often found in furniture polishes.

The pastes should be applied to the floor with a cleaning rag in a thin, even coat to within 22–30 cm of the skirting board as the buffing will carry enough polish over the floor edge where there is little or no wear, and so prevent excessive build up of the wax. The paste should be left for a few minutes before buffing to a shine with a clean, soft cloth or left about 15–20 minutes before buffing with an electric polisher. The surface may thus be kept in good condition by sweeping, mopping or vacuum cleaning and buffing, repolishing only when necessary. Too much polish should be avoided as this will mean extra work in buffing and may leave a slippery surface. Any 'build up' of wax should be removed periodically by rubbing the floor with fine steel wool or a nylon web pad, dipped in white spirit and immediately wiping up the loosened wax and dirt with a damp cloth—the floor should then be repolished.

The liquid spirit based polishes may contain as much as 90% spirit solvent and they should be applied thinly over the floor by hand or machine and buffed to a shine in similar manner to the paste polishes. Any 'build up' of wax should be similarly avoided.

Both paste and liquid spirit based polishes may be used on wood, cork and linoleum (but more often now treated with water based polishes) floorings as well as wooden furniture and walls, but they harm thermoplastic (asphalt based tiles), rubber and asphalt composition floorings.

2 *Water based floor polishes* also consist of blends of waxes but natural waxes are tending to be replaced by resins. They contain no spirit solvents but consist of a colloidal suspension of waxes or synthetic resins in water and are always liquid. Some of the earlier 'no-buff' emulsion formulations do not prove very satisfactory under heavy wear conditions producing a brittle, slippery and powdery finish. Newer formulations are based on acrylic, polyethylene or vinyl polymers and give an increased water resistance, gloss and toughness.

Into the polymer formulation a complex of metallic elements may be incorporated shielding the breakpoints in the polymer chain against the penetration of detergent solutions and liquid stains. The finish is therefore tough, and wash and stain resistant and is known as a *metallised finish or polish*.

As these water based polishes contain no spirit solvent they have no cleaning properties. They should be applied to a perfectly clean floor because extraneous materials may affect their performance. In use, the water evaporates, leaving a hard continuous film which in many cases dries shiny and requires no buffing. Periodically, any 'build up' of polish should be removed with very hot water and a special synthetic detergent formulated for polish removal, and the floor repolished when dry.

Where the floor area is sufficiently large to enable the use of a polishing machine *spray buffing* may be used to repair the emulsion coating as wear and damage dictate (i.e. instead of repolishing). The emulsion is diluted and a small quantity of detergent is added. This mixture is sprayed lightly on to the floor area requiring it and the sprayed sections are buffed to dryness. (It is possible to use proprietary spray buffing formulations in aerosols.) To ensure uniformity of appearance adjoining areas can be dry buffed with the same pad. It is essential that after spray buffing the floor is dry mopped to pick up any residue. The dilution of the emulsion avoids any machine drag and build up of the polish. The elimination of scuff marks, scratches and signs of wear is brought about by the re-emulsifying action of the spray and the tendency for the heat from the pad friction and the weight of the machine to 'melt' the surface of the emulsion polish. Properly carried out there should be no 'build up' in lighter traffic areas or along the floor edges—routine spray buffing may save time and money in floor maintenance. Spray buffing is not a method of cleaning a dirty floor. Dust and tracked-on soil should first be removed by sweeping, dust or damp mopping and spray buffing is only suitable when the flooring is protected with a good coating (2–3 thin coats) of polymer finish and should be followed by mopping the floor.

During spray buffing there is a possibility of dirt being carried into the synthetic finish during the re-emulsifying action of the spray. Because of this some people prefer *spray cleaning* to spray buffing, when a dilute solution of a neutral detergent (e.g. 1 in 60) is sprayed over the polymer finish and buffed until dry.

Water based polishes may be used on thermoplastic, rubber, vinyl, or linoleum floorings as well as sealed wood and sealed cork.

Owing to the water based polishes drying to a shiny finish they are often confused with floor seals. The latter are not polishes, but are semi-permanent finishes, of cellulosic or plastic composition, applied to render the floor impermeable and to protect its surface (see Chapter 7).

Furniture polishes consist of special blends of waxes and spirit solvents and may be paste, liquid or of a cream consistency.

There are also 'spray on' wax polishes for furniture, and these contain a high silicone content and require no buffing, but they are expensive and may be wasteful, if not used carefully.

Furniture polishes are intended for use on wooden furniture and walls, and provided they have not a high silicone content when they are too slippery, they can be used on wood, linoleum and cork floors. The liquid or cream polishes may be used on leather.

Paste wax furniture polishes now frequently include silicones to give a harder and more lasting shine, to improve the resistance to heat, moisture and sunlight and to make the polish easier to spread. The polish should be applied sparingly with a soft cloth and rubbed up well when the spirit evaporates and leaves a thin layer of wax and these layers over a period of time give a high gloss. These polishes are particularly suitable for antiques and other pieces of furniture where the shine is dependent on the layers of wax. Too much polish must not be applied at any one time or a sticky finish will result.

Cream wax polishes are emulsions of a blend of light coloured waxes and solvents with or without silicones. There is less wax than in the paste polishes and the greater proportion of solvents gives some cleaning action. They may be applied with a damp cloth and rubbed up immediately and are suitable for most types of furniture remembering that the build-up in the layers of wax will be slower than with paste polishes.

Liquid no-rub polishes have a high percentage of solvent giving some cleaning action. They are good for the removal of food stains, drink rings and finger marks. They are applied with a soft cloth, when they dry to a haze in a few minutes and result in a shine when this is wiped off. These polishes are most suitable for furniture which already has a shine, e.g. French polished furniture.

Spray-on polishes are similar to the no-rub polishes, but there is some alteration in the solvents used which necessitates that the surface should be wiped immediately with a soft cloth and the polish not left to dry. These polishes may be sprayed directly on to dusty surfaces enabling dusting, cleaning and polishing to be combined in one operation. They may also be used on glass surfaces, chrome and ceramic tiles, etc. For economical use the polish may be sprayed on to the cloth for polishing small areas.

Shoe polishes are manufactured with the cleaning of leather shoes in mind (no polish is required for shoes made of plastic), and consist of special blends of waxes, spirit solvents and dyes, and may be paste, cream or liquid. As with other wax polishes, the spirit evaporates leaving a film of wax which is waterproof, and can be rubbed to a shine.

The polish should be applied to shoes free of dust and mud, worked into the shoe surface with a brush, and rubbed to a shine with a polishing brush and soft cloth.

Impregnated paper shoe shiners are frequently provided in hotels.

Metal polishes consist basically of a fine abrasive, which when rubbed on to the surface removes the tarnish, resulting from the attack on the metal by certain compounds in the air and some foodstuffs. In the liquid polishes, the abrasive is mixed with a grease solvent, and in some cases an acid to help in the removal of the tarnish, and the production of a shine. The polish is applied with rag, or with wadding already impregnated with polish, and the article is then rubbed up with a soft, dry rag.

Metals react differently to the various cleaning materials, so the exact composition of the polish will depend on the metal for which the polish is intended. The most frequently cleaned metals are brass, copper (hard metal) and silver and silver plate (soft metal) so in the main there are two types of metal polishes, one for the hard metals and the other for the soft. Pewter is sometimes polished, and then either type may be used. Chromium and stainless steel should not need polishing, but there are special polishes available when necessary. Aluminium, tin and zinc are not normally polished; iron and steel, because they rust easily, are generally given a protective coating of enamel or zinc (galvanised iron) or nylon (dipped in a bath of liquid nylon), when no polishing is required. Copper and brass may be lacquered and aluminium anodised, when they will all resist tarnishing.

Hard metals when very tarnished may be cleaned by rubbing with an acid, generally lemon or vinegar; a fine abrasive is added to the acid and this is the basis for copper pickle used in large kitchens for cleaning copper pans. The acid must be washed off quickly or further staining will result. This method removes stains but produces no shine, so ornamental brass and copper are polished afterwards.

Silver and silver plate may be cleaned with various polishes used in liquid form and based on precipitated whiting and jewellers' rouge, for instance proprietary silver polishes, plate powder mixed with methylated spirit, ammonia or water and 'long term' silver polish. The latter as it cleans, leaves a film bonded to the silver which resists tarnishing for a considerable time. Each of these may be applied with a rag and rubbed off when dry to produce a shine.

In addition to silver polishes, there are certain cleansers which will remove stains and tarnish but which do not produce a shine, e.g. (1) an acid solution of a thiourea compound (the basis of silver dips) into which the articles are dipped and then washed, and (2) a hot soda solution to which a sheet of aluminium and the silver have been added when a chemical exchange process takes place and this is the Polivit method.

N.B. Silver may also be cleaned in a burnishing machine (see Chapter 15).

Housekeeping Stores

From the previously mentioned cleaning agents the *housekeeper* will choose the ones most suitable for her establishment and after the original issue to the maids, replenishments will be required from time to time when the rule of 'new for old' and 'full for empty' may be applied or there may be a 'topping up' system.

In some establishments there is one large main store run by a storekeeper and the housekeeping stores are issued from it to the individual maid or cleaner at set times. In other places the maids make out their own requisition lists and hand these in for the *housekeeper* to countersign and the items are collected from the stores by a porter and taken to the maids. In this way the *housekeeper* has a better idea of the amounts being issued to her department and the maids do not waste time collecting their stores.

Yet another way of obtaining stores is from a conveniently situated housekeeping store cupboard kept under lock and key, and the responsibility for it is given to one of the assistant housekeepers and maids come at set times of the day for renewals or replenishments. In the case of the 'topping up' system, the *housekeeper* or storekeeper will make the necessary arrangements for restocking.

Powdered items may be bought in bulk and this involves the issuing of small quantities into suitable containers, when it is possible with careless handling for wastage and mess to occur. Paste polishes may also be bought in bulk, but this necessitates stirring from time to time as the spirit rises to the surface, and this can be tiresome. Liquid detergents are frequently bought in large containers with a special pouring device, and this means the provision of bottles for issuing individual amounts. So, although there may be an economy of money when buying in large quantities, wastage of materials can occur, and there is much more time involved in the issuing of broken quantities. All containers should be clearly labelled. New types of cleaning agents should always be well tried out in small quantities before a bulk order is placed.

Toilet paper is ordered by the gross, and often arrangements are made for deliveries to come automatically, unless otherwise requested. When ordering, the type of fitment must be remembered and these may be for inter-leaved or roll type paper. The paper may be thin and smooth or soft tissue, and in many instances both kinds are provided in the same toilet.

In all cases involving storage, rotation of stock should be practised, and items which are little used should obviously be bought in smaller quantities.

The actual buying of the items in any establishment may be done
through the head office of a group;
by a buyer;
by a responsible storekeeper;
by the *housekeeper*.

Where the items are indented from a main store, a stock list kept by the *housekeeper* is not so important, but where deliveries are made direct to the housekeeping department, a much more careful check of stock is necessary, in order to prevent waste and running out of stock. The frequency with which stock is taken varies from establishment to establishment.

Where items are bought in bulk, unless there are large scales, actual stock cannot be taken, so in a housekeeping store the stock of these items is an estimated amount.

Part of a Stores sheet could be:

Item	Unit	Stock in hand	Re-ceipts	Total	Less issues	Book stock	Actual stock	Discrep-ancies
Liquid detergent	litres							
Powdered detergent	kg.							
Scouring powder	tins							
Floor polish	tins							
Dusters	each							

In addition to the cleaning cloths and agents there will be other items required in the department for the use of the guests or staff especially in hotels. The following is a list of some of these items which may be kept in the housekeeping stores:

toilet soap
toilet paper
drawer lining paper
writing paper
coat hangers
disclaimer notices
laundry and dry cleaning
     lists
ash trays
spare electric light bulbs
candles
electric blankets
electric razors ⎫
electric tooth ⎬ for hire
   brushes   ⎭

book matches
paper tissues
small containers of detergents
impregnated paper shoe shiners
brochures
'do not disturb' cards
tooth glasses
hot water bottles
bedpan and urine bottle
other accessories put into
     guests' rooms according to
     house custom (guests' supplies).

A small supply of toothbrushes (including those for electric holders), toothpaste, face flannels and feminine towels may be kept for sale to guests when required.

Maids' Service Room

A service room or pantry is the place from which a maid works, where she keeps her equipment (generally marked with her name, number of the floor or section), cleaning agents and other necessities for her work. She may share the room with one or more other maids and when their work is finished the door should be locked. The room should be easily cleaned, with as few things on the floor as possible.

In an hotel when the routine work is finished, the maid sits in this room and is on call until she goes off duty. Depending on the establishment early morning tea may be served from this room, a store of linen kept, (sufficient to re-sheet the section or sections), hot water bottles filled, cloths washed and dried and when necessary slops emptied and chambers cleaned. Thus in all establishments some or all of the following articles may be provided:

a sink with running water and a draining board;
a floor sink, similar to a shower tray with the taps so positioned that buckets and other containers (e.g. floor mopping and scrubbing equipment) can be filled and emptied easily;
electric or gas water boiler, or large kettle with some means of heating it;

table and chair;
cupboard or shelves for early morning tea-trays and china;
cupboard for floor linen stock;
rail for drying tea towels and dusters;
storage space for cleaning equipment and cleaning agents;
rubbish bin or disposable paper sack;
space for maid's trolley if used.

Cleaning Methods

Any establishment has to present an inviting, clean and well cared for appearance at all times, and the cleaning should be carried out at a time when it will cause as little inconvenience as possible. Thus the public rooms and offices are cleaned by maids before breakfast when there is less activity. In some establishments, the public rooms are cleaned during the night by the night porter when only the final dusting is left for the maids, or by contract cleaners. During the day the lounge is normally looked after by the lounge waiter or one of the uniformed staff regarding papers, ashtrays and cushions etc. and the housekeeper inspects the area at intervals.

There is little work that can be done 'on the floors' before breakfast, other than calls and the serving of early morning teas; corridors and staircases are not normally cleaned before breakfast in case *guests* might be disturbed, and maids should realise that noise, e.g. shouting, raucous laughter, the banging of equipment and the clatter of crockery, must be avoided at all times. *Guests* should be inconvenienced as little as possible, and their belongings should only be moved when necessary. Drawers should not be opened by a maid in an occupied room, but clothes may be hung in the wardrobe. On no account should a maid try on jewellery or make use of any of the *guests'* personal belongings such as cosmetics. Newspapers, unless in the wastepaper basket, should not be thrown away.

It is customary for maids to leave the door ajar while they are working in a room (this gives the appearance that everything is above board), and owing to the door normally being opposite the window, care should be taken to avoid articles being blown off the dressing table by the curtain. Equipment and cleaning agents should not be left untidily in the corridor for people to trip over, nor should they ever be placed on the bed or upholstered furniture, and where it is used, a trolley outside the door indicates that the maid is in the room. In some hotels, there may be a 'maid finder' device outside each door, and the maid operates this to denote that she is in the room.

The cleaning of rooms falls into three categories: a daily clean; a special clean; a spring clean.

Rooms in use require a daily clean so that they give a comfortable and presentable appearance.

After some days' use rooms will require a more thorough clean when extra jobs are added to the daily routine and this is a special clean.

A spring clean is a very thorough clean carried out annually; in a seasonal establishment when it is closed and in other places at convenient times depending on occupancy.

In order to help maids in their work and the *housekeeper* in training them, it is possible for orders of work, incorporating work simplification, to be planned. It is a simple matter to plan an order of work for cleaning a specific article, e.g. a wash basin, but difficulties arise when it comes to rooms as they vary so much, in addition to the fact that they may be occupied or vacant.

In general it should be remembered that

sweeping with a broom is done before dusting, and dusting before vacuum cleaning;

daily dusting is done from high to low;

vertical surfaces need dusting occasionally from stretch level;

bending with stiff knees should be avoided;

where there are alternative methods of cleaning the least harmful ones should be used;

cleaning methods while being efficient should be economical of time, labour and cleaning materials.

The following are suggested orders of work for the cleaning of several articles and different types of rooms, but it must be stressed that there will in all probability be adjustments necessary in differing circumstances, and that orders of work are not necessarily the *methods* by which cleaning should be done. Before starting the work it is expected that maids will have been instructed regarding the necessary 'tools' for the job.

N.B. Only a few articles are mentioned here and others are covered in their respective chapters.

To Clean a Telephone
1 Dust daily and wipe ear piece free of grease.
2 Occasionally clean the dial and disinfect ear and mouthpiece.

To Deal with a TV set
1 Remove plug from wall to disconnect electricity.
2 Move set as little as possible.
3 Dust all over.
4 Use damp cloth to clean screen.
5 Report frayed flexes and other defects.

The Care of an Electric Blanket
1 Remove plug from wall to disconnect electricity.

2 Keep blanket as flat as possible, not crumpled up or bent unduly.
3 Avoid getting wet.
4 When necessary, send protective covering to the laundry.
5 Report frayed flexes and other defects.
(N.B. Electric blankets should be serviced regularly.)

To Clean Mirrors and Glass Surfaces
1 Dust daily.
2 Wipe with damp cloth when necessary.
3 Polish with lint-free cloth.
4 Treat frame according to kind.
(N.B. Hair spray marks can be removed with a cloth moistened with methylated spirit.)

To Clean Bathmats (other than launderable ones)
Cork
1 Wipe daily with a damp cloth.
2 When necessary, wash and rub using fine scouring powder.
3 Rinse and stand upright to dry.
(N.B. Cork on the seat of a W.C. or stool should be cleaned similarly.)
Rubber
1 Wipe daily with a damp cloth.
2 When necessary, wash and rub using fine scouring powder.
3 Rinse and dry.
(N.B. A rubber mat round the W.C. pedestal should be treated similarly.)

Lavatory basins (wash basins) are still predominantly made of vitreous china usually of white or a pale colour, and the surface is non-porous and very smooth. For hygienic reasons this smooth surface should remain intact, and therefore care must be taken to prevent chipping, cracking or scratching, as any of these will make the surface more difficult to clean, and more susceptible to staining. Dripping taps should be reported for maintenance as soon as possible or a hard water stain results, and when this occurs it should be removed with a weak acid, e.g. vinegar or a cut lemon, and if this is not effective a stronger acid such as oxalic may be used under the supervision of the *housekeeper*. There are also proprietary substances sold for the removal of hard water marks. After the use of an acid the surface must be rinsed thoroughly or the acid will harm the glaze.

Brass taps are not frequently found these days but where they are they require cleaning with a metal polish; chromium plated taps, chains and plugholes need no polishing but merely rubbing with a damp cloth.

Every wash basin normally has an overflow and this, as well as the plug, plughole and soapwell must be kept free from dried soap, scum and fluff.

Wash basins may be on a pedestal or be cantilevered, and these parts as well as the mirror, shelf and surround need attention during cleaning of the basin.

To Clean a Lavatory Basin
1 Remove hair, fluff, etc., from waste, chain and overflow.
2 Wash and dry toothglass.
3 Clean basin and surrounds with swab and fine abrasive paying particular attention to base of taps.
4 Rub up taps and dry basin.

Baths are made of enamelled iron, vitreous china, fibre glass or perspex. In many establishments there are showers used in conjunction with baths, necessitating extra fittings and shower curtains or screens.

Baths are cleaned in a similar manner to wash basins including the surround, but there is more likelihood of scum and staining making cleaning more difficult.

If there is a shower, the fittings and curtain rail should be cleaned; the curtains should be wiped and left hanging inside the bath.

Water closets are made of vitreous china while the seat and lid are normally made of plastic; the pan may be on a pedestal clamped to the floor or it may be cantilevered, and in conjunction with it there is a water cistern (water waste preventer).

The W.C. pan requires the same care as the basin and bath, in that it must not become scratched. The W.C. pan becomes easily stained and requires regular and thorough brushing with a lavatory (toilet) brush. Toilet cleansers which are acidic are available and may be used when brushing is insufficient. If it becomes badly stained, the water in the trap should be removed and a fine abrasive used with friction, or even concentrated hydrochloric acid may be used *under strict supervision*, and this is a job more for the maintenance department than for the housekeeping staff.

To Clean a W.C.
1 Flush pan, brush well and flush again.
2 If pan is still stained, use toilet cleanser.
3 Brush and flush again.
4 Wipe pedestal, seat and lid with a suitable cloth, and dry.
5 Check for toilet paper and leave a spare.

A **bidet** is made of vitreous china and has chromium plated fittings. There is a tendency for staining by hard water and a bidet is cleaned similarly to a wash basin.

All or some of the above may be housed in a **bathroom** and there may be other fittings and furniture such as a sanibin, stool, towel rail, etc. which should be cleaned according to their kind. In addition there are other surfaces, e.g. shelves and walls and these show soiling from condensation and dust, especially talcum powder and so need to be cleaned with a damp cloth. The floor should be of some easily cleaned material which may be washed daily.

For further details concerning bathrooms see p. 223.

Daily Cleaning of a Bathroom with tiled walls and floor
1 Remove soiled linen and empty sanibin.
2 Clean W.C.
3 Clean bath, shower and wash basin.
4 Wipe remaining fittings and surfaces.
5 Put out clean towels and bathmat. Check for soap, toilet paper, lavatory cloth and paper bags for sanitary towels.
6 Wash the floor.

In the past a **pedestal cupboard** was provided in all bedrooms for the storage of the chamber and the contents of the chambers were carried in a slop pail to a housemaid's sink (or to a toilet) to be emptied. The chamber had to be washed and dried and the pedestal cupboard kept clean and pleasant smelling. One of the more serious omissions a maid and an assistant housekeeper could make, was to forget to check the contents of the pedestal cupboard.

Nowadays chambers are not provided in bedrooms unless specifically requested and when they have been used the covered chamber is carried and emptied in a toilet.

Bed making

This constitutes a large proportion of the room maids' work in hotels and similar establishments, and a badly made bed can upset the guest and the appearance of the room. An unmade bed gives a room an unkempt appearance, so beds are made as early as possible, and unless some thought is given to the method a great deal of time and energy can be wasted. The maid may walk round the bed many times unless she is taught to conserve her energy.

To make a bed
strip the clothes from the bed on to a chair and leave to air;
turn mattress occasionally, unless made of latex or plastic foam;
replace under-blanket;
put on bottom sheet, right side up and tuck in all round, making a mitre at all four corners—
To mitre a corner: tuck in along the foot or head of the mattress, lift

flap of sheet from a point along the side about 30 cm from the corner, and tuck in remaining portion, drop flap and tuck in:

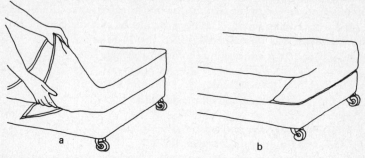

To show a mitred corner: (a) in the process of being made   (b) completed

put on top sheet, wrong side up, to reach just beyond the head of the mattress;

put on blankets separately, to reach just short of the top sheet;

put on quilt if used;

mitre one bottom corner and turn over sufficient of the sheet and blankets at the top to leave a space for the pillows, approximately 60 cm;

tuck in that side; repeat on other side;

replace the pillows with open ends away from the door;

put on bedspread.

For further details of beds and beddings see Chapter 10.

There are other methods of bedmaking according to house custom and some of these incorporate 'turning down' during the initial bedmaking process.

'Turning down' in the evening is an increasingly expensive process owing to labour costs and full 'night service' i.e. complete turning down, is being practised less and less but it is still to be expected in luxury hotels.

One method of turning down a bed:

remove and fold bedspread and put in a convenient place;

untuck part of one side of the bedclothes and fold back the clothes to form a right-angled triangle;

neaten the edges by folding under surplus bedding and tuck in at the side;

place night attire on the bed, dressing gown on a chair and slippers at the foot of the chair.

N.B. It is usual to turn down the side of the bed nearer the dressing table and if there are twin beds the two inside edges.

There are other methods and opinions regarding the turning down of beds, and it should be remembered that studio type beds often involve more work on the part of the maid.

When 'turning down' it is assumed that a maid will carry out the following work, as well as the actual turning down of the bed;

> empty any litter from ashtrays and wastepaper basket, and generally tidy the room;
> wipe the bath and wash basin, paying particular attention to the toothglass;
> fold the towels;
> check the lights;
> adjust the windows, draw the curtains and later maybe put in hot water bottles or switch on electric blankets.

The service of early morning tea in hotels and clubs

In some hotels early morning teas are served by floor waiters, while in others there are tea making facilities in the rooms (comfort trays), but often room-maids carry out this duty from their service rooms. A tea book is made up by the night porter, and a list is given to the room-maid when she comes on duty early in the morning, and to this list she adds any extra teas that she may serve in order that the charge may be put on the guests' bills. Each maid has a small stock of tea and sugar which

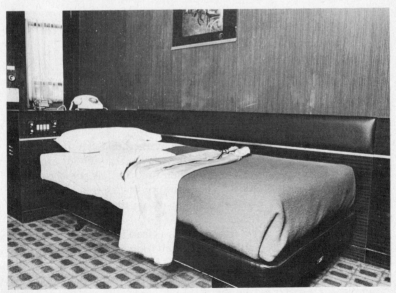

A bed turned down for the night

is replenished daily according to her list, but milk is fetched each morning from the stillroom or kitchen. In some hotels the night porter may have the water boiling in the maid's service room to enable her to make tea straight away if necessary, and any teas requested before the roommaid comes on duty will be dealt with by him.

The trays are often kept laid up in the service room ready for use after the crockery has been washed up. The tea spoons which have a habit of disappearing are carefully guarded by the room-maid and either cleaned by her or taken occasionally to the plate room.

For the service of early morning tea, the room-maid:

1 Knocks on the door and if no reply, waits a few seconds, knocks again and enters.
2 If dark, switches on the light.
3 Says 'good morning' cheerfully.
4 Places tray on bedside table with newspapers if ordered.
5 Makes sure guest is awake.
6 Draws curtains if requested.
7 Closes the door gently.

In some hotels the maids are responsible for floor service throughout the day, and in this case it is usual for the prepared tray and food to come direct from the kitchen, where the 'dirties' are sent back and the room-maid is not concerned with the washing-up.

There are certain general procedures for cleaning any room and a very simple *order of work for any area* could be:-

1 Open windows where possible.
2 Remove litter and dirty crockery, etc.
3 Attend to main jobs, bed, fireplace, etc.
4 Sweep if required.
5 Dust and if necessary mop.
6 Vacuum clean.
7 Survey the room.

A *daily routine* is normally carried out by the maid on one visit to a room but in some instances she may do one job throughout a number of rooms e.g. stripping the beds and then the next job and so on until the work is completed. This cleaning routine (block cleaning) is more suited to establishments where it is known that the rooms are likely to be empty for at least all the morning.

It is usual to give a *special* or *more thorough* clean to all rooms from time to time when occupied, and also to vacated rooms before reletting. This entails extra attention being given to such items as carpet edges, upholstery, furniture, and paintwork. As with the daily routine this special clean may be carried out by the maid on one visit to a room as would be required in a vacated room, or it may be more convenient to add one or two jobs to the daily routine so completing the special clean within a few days.

The cleaning of a private sitting-room or lounge

This is one of the jobs a maid does before breakfast, bearing in mind that she must be very quiet and possibly not use the vacuum cleaner. The work that she will do in this room is removing rubbish, straightening chairs, bunching up cushions, etc., dusting; if necessary the carpet can be dealt with later in the day.

The contents of the sideboard and/or cocktail cabinet in a guest's room are not the concern of the room-maid, but of the floor waiter.

The cleaning of staircases

Stairs may be close carpeted, or the carpet may only cover about two-thirds of the stair in which case there are two surfaces to clean. By using suitable attachments to a vacuum cleaner the two surfaces and skirting board may be cleaned together.

In the case of uncarpeted stairs, they should be swept daily and washed and/or scrubbed according to the material, when necessary. If a staircase has to be scrubbed while people are using it, then provided that it is wide enough, half should be done at a time, enabling the people to walk up and down on the dry part of the staircase.

It should be remembered that where the side of any staircase is open, dust and dirt may fall through, and so, when sweeping, the dirt should be swept towards the wall on each step.

All bannisters and handrails should be dusted before vacuum cleaning, or after sweeping, and washed or polished occasionally according to material.

Stair rods of brass or polished wood may still be used, but nowadays the stair carpet may be held firmly in position by the use of the 'tackless gripper' (see p. 154) which eliminates the use of rods and makes cleaning much easier.

The cleaning of the lifts is rarely the concern of the houskeeper but is usually the work of the uniformed staff.

The cleaning of utility rooms or kitchen/dining areas in hostels (amenity areas)

In hostels and halls of residence the cleaning of kitchen/dining areas for the use of residents follows the normal cleaning process but the area does present problems for the cleaner.

In a given kitchen/dining area there will be a refrigerator and food storage cupboards and these are the responsibility of the users, as well as the washing up. The cleaner, therefore, cleans the area including the sinks, draining boards and cookers. However, problems arise when the sink is full of dirty crockery and the cooker has been carelessly used and more than the allotted time is needed for cleaning.

Order of work for the daily clean of an occupied room *with a wash basin and carpet square*

1 Open window, if necessary remove early morning tea or breakfast tray.
2 Strip bed.
3 Empty ashtrays, waste-paper basket and generally tidy room.
4 Make bed.
5 Attend to wash basin; fold towels and check for soap.
6 Adjust window.
7 Dust all furniture and fittings.
8 Mop surround.
9 Carpet sweep or vacuum clean carpet square.
10 Survey room and close door.

Order of work for the special cleaning of a vacated room, *close carpeted and with a private bathroom*

1 Open the window, if necessary remove early morning tea or break-fast tray.
2 Check for lost property and clean drawers, inside of wardrobe and check for coathangers.
3 Strip the bed, remove soiled linen including towels.
4 Empty ashtrays, waste-paper basket, etc.
5 Make bed with clean linen.
6 Adjust window.
7 Sweep carpet edges and upholstery if no vacuum cleaner attachments.
8 Dust all furniture and fittings, polishing if necessary; remove marks from paintwork and attend to mirrors, telephone, TV, radio and lights.
9 Attend to the bathroom—
   Wash basin, bath, W.C. (see p. 44).
   Wipe or dust all surfaces.
   Put out clean towels, soap and toilet paper.
   Clean floor according to kind.
10 Vacuum clean upholstery and carpet edges if suitable attachments.
11 Vacuum clean carpet.

12 Survey rooms and close door.

An alternative method is to clean the bathroom while the bed is being aired and ideally the assistant housekeeper should have checked the vacated room for lost property, maintenance and missing articles before the entry of the maid.

Annual or Spring Cleaning

As far as the housekeeper is concerned, spring cleaning has to be carried out in all areas of her department. The spring cleaning of a lounge has obviously to be done at a quiet time of the year, and sometimes parts of the work are done during the night such as carpet shampooing and paintwashing. In most places, there will be off or quiet periods, and the annual cleaning will be carried out during these times. It is usual for a number of rooms to be 'taken off' together and the annual clean is often carried out in conjunction with redecoration or alteration of a room, or more often, a floor of rooms. As it is a combined operation involving the housekeeping and maintenance departments, the work will be planned between them and such items as new furniture, carpets and other furnishings required in the reassembling of the room must be planned well ahead. As soon as it is known that rooms are to be taken 'off', the reception office must be notified.

When annual cleaning a room it should be remembered that all

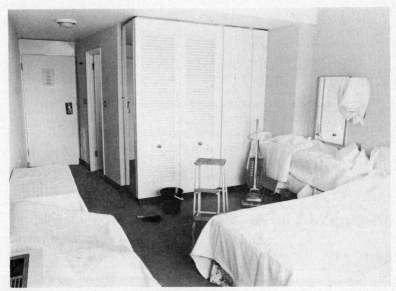

A room in the process of being spring-cleaned

launderable linen will go to the laundry, and all loose furnishings and bedding will go to the dry cleaners or laundry, or be shaken, folded and put aside until required. A fitted carpet will be completely covered by druggets and shampooed later. A carpet square will be taken up after being marked to enable it to be turned round when relaying to even wear and maybe shampooed.

To prevent indentations and possible rust marks on a damp carpet, small pieces of plastic material will be placed under the legs of furniture.

During the preliminary preparation, repairs of all kinds whether to furniture, floors, plumbing or electrical fittings, will be noted and either dealt with *in situ* or the articles removed to be repaired elsewhere.

In an hotel, house porters or valet-porters will help the maids with some of the jobs done during spring cleaning.

Order of work for annual cleaning a bedroom

1 Ventilate room.
2 Strip bed and deal accordingly with linen and bedding.
3 Remove loose furnishings.
4 Vacuum clean bed and upholstered furniture.
5 Place cleaned small articles including lamp shades, on bed and cover.
6 Vacuum clean, then cover or take up carpet.
7 Wipe or wash furniture inside and out.
8 Stack and cover furniture or remove from room.
   The room can now be redecorated or washed down. If no redecoration:
9 Sweep walls and floor.
10 Wash paintwork and have windows cleaned.
11 Thoroughly clean wash basin.
12 Wash floor if necessary and leave to dry.
13 Have carpet relaid or uncovered and vacuum clean it.
14 Have curtains rehung.
15 Reline drawers, polish furniture and if necessary reposition it.
16 Uncover bed, remove small articles and put in place.
17 Have carpets shampooed.
18 Make bed with clean linen and bedding.
19 If there is a surround, mop and polish it.
20 Finally dust, mop if necessary and vacuum clean carpet.
21 Survey room and close door.

Coverage

The hours a housekeeping department is manned will vary considerably and will be determined by the areas to be maintained by the department and the type of service to be given. Not only will these factors influence the organisation of the department as far as coverage is concerned but they will, of course, have a bearing on the number of staff and the amount of work that can be undertaken by each employee (see p. 266).

The type of service offered to the *guest* is a question of house policy and/or economics, and the housekeeping department must be geared to meet the demands made on it.

In hotels and similar establishments the guests pay for service and the hours the housekeeping department is manned must cover not only the time taken for the actual cleaning of the areas to be maintained, but to enable the service to be given to the guests as and when it becomes necessary. The hours of coverage may therefore appear lengthy, but it is necessary that someone is available at the most likely times to meet the guests' demands.

In university halls of residence, nurses' homes, etc., the residents do not receive the same amount of personal service as guests in hotels and the housekeeping staff are more concerned with keeping a reasonable standard of cleanliness at the lowest possible cost; these places are therefore staffed for cleaning and once this is completed there is not the same need for the housekeeping department to be manned.

It is possible of course, that in any establishment there is work which can only be carried out by day and other work which is more conveniently done in the evening. There will be, therefore, tremendous variations in the hours covered by the housekeeping staff, not only from one type of establishment to another but within a group of similar establishments.

Since the housekeeping wages bill accounts for a large part of the cleaning costs it needs to be kept as low as possible and the housekeeper has to employ only the minimum number of staff. In some places it has been found more practicable to employ part-time staff (women who work four to five hours in the morning and possibly others who work two to three hours in the evening), but it should be remembered that two lots of insurance stamps may be needed and the casual hourly rate of pay is higher than that for a full time maid.

Hotels' Staff Duties

In an hotel an average coverage may be from 7 a.m. to 10 p.m. However, there are hotels where the staff start and finish at other times, earlier or later and even give a 24-hour service, while in the small hotels there may be times at which there are no housekeeping staff on duty and any queries will be dealt with by the general assistant, manageress or manager.

The busiest times in the housekeeping department are in the mornings when resheeting and essential cleaning of the rooms is being dealt with. This work cannot normally be commenced before about 8.30 or 9 a.m. but some of the room-maids may have started their duty before this to serve the early morning teas. There are hotels where early morning teas are not served by the housekeeping staff but by floor waiters, or there may be tea making facilities in the rooms and in such places maids may come in at 8 to 8.30 a.m. rather than the earlier hour of 7 a.m.

Where maids 'turn down', draw corridor curtains and are on call to attend to guests' requirements, evenings may also be a busy time but there are hotels where no 'turning down' is done in the evening. In these hotels there will be a minimum of maids on duty to deal with unexpected and late departures and, in the case of Post Houses and Motor Hotels, rooms being let more than once in 24 hours. There are also hotels where no maids are on duty in the evening and requests and complaints from guests will be dealt with by the housekeeper if on duty or by the receptionist.

The afternoons are for completing the morning's work and carrying out extra jobs allocated by the housekeeper.

In some hotels guests spend a lot of time in their rooms, having breakfast in bed, resting in the afternoon, changing leisurely in the evening, and requiring the odd needle and cotton, flower vases, the use of the iron and board, etc., and this impedes the work of the room-maid, and so in these hotels maids will be given a smaller section to service, and when they are not actually working they will be in their service rooms on call.

There are other hotels geared to business people, where the rooms are of the studio type, and the guests may have business associates or friends **in their rooms at any period of the day**; this may mean that the guests will ask for the room to be serviced by a particular time, and if there are several such requests this may present difficulties for the maid.

In still other hotels and particularly transit hotels, there will be many guests staying only one night, who arrive late and leave early, and so require practically no personal service; other guests who though they may stay longer, spend little time in their rooms, and thus in these hotels the room-maid's work will be very straightforward and without many interruptions. Package tours may disrupt the work because of their arrival or departure at awkward hours and rooms may have to be serviced quickly for new arrivals.

So, in any hotel there will be one maid per section where possible in the mornings, and in the evenings the numbers will depend on the type of hotel, and one maid may deal with one or several sections. In order that the essential servicing of rooms can be carried out in the mornings and evenings, some split duties may be necessary, but as they are unpopular, especially with non-resident maids, as few split duties as possible should be given. According to the Catering Wages Order, maids whose work is spread over more than twelve hours, are entitled to extra pay, unless their current wage already exceeds the regulation minimum plus the extra allowances. Arrangements for a 5 day week are made where possible,.in some cases the two days off being taken together and in others not.

The room-maid

The tendency today is for room-maids to service a section of approximately 10–15 rooms, with private bathrooms, and maybe including the corridor, without any help from a housemaid or cleaner. This work is of great importance because it contributes to the comfort of the guest and hence his impression of the hotel. It involves a knowledge and use of social and technical skills which should have been explained to them during their periods of training under the housekeeper or training officer. Room-maids are responsible to the assistant housekeepers who by supervision of them and the checking of their rooms ensure an accepted standard in the hotel.

Punctuality, neat appearance, courtesy and the anticipation of the needs of others are essential qualities in the maid. She needs to work quickly and efficiently following the housekeeper's instructions regarding methods of cleaning and cleaning programmes. As well as this she needs to plan herself in order that vacated rooms are serviced before occupied, that guests' requests for their rooms to be serviced at a certain time are met with and that economies are practised with regard to time, labour and the use of materials.

She needs to work quietly and tidily causing as little inconvenience to the guest as possible. The handling of guests' and hotel property should be such that no damage is done to the articles and nothing is thrown away without the certainty that it is rubbish. The maid should be fully aware of the need for safety and security within the department, avoiding any action which may lead to an accident or a fire hazard. She should understand the necessity for the strict control of keys and she should

keep them on her person;

never use them to let a stranger into a room;

always hand them in at the end of a duty period according to house custom;

hand in to the housekeeper any keys found left in doors or lying around.

To help the housekeeper and the smoother running of the hotel the maid should realise the importance of reporting promptly such things as:

room occupancy;

lost property;

light luggage;

missing or damaged articles;

anything in need of repair;

anything of a suspicious nature;

illness of a guest;

accidents;

anything for which a charge should be made on a guest's bill e.g. early morning teas, dogs in rooms, etc.

In order to do her work satisfactorily she requires to be told of relevant details for her section as early as possible, e.g. departures, requirements for new guests. This information will be given to her by the assistant housekeeper as soon as the latter has received it from the receptionist, initially by means of the Arrivals and Departures list and later by telephone or other means of communication between the housekeeper and receptionist.

The hours that a room-maid may work vary a great deal and for some it may be a straight shift of 8 hours for 5 days a week, and assuming the maids serve early morning teas they may work 7 a.m.–3.30 p.m. If they do not serve early morning teas then they may not come on until 8 or 8.30 a.m.

If in the above cases 'turning down' is done in the evening separate maids would be engaged for such hours as 5–10 p.m. There would be fewer maids than in the morning as they would be expected to service larger sections. However 'turning down' is much less prevalent than it used to be and so there are places where only 1 or 2 maids are on in the evening to service late and extra departures and carry out any other necessary jobs, and in others there may be no maids on at all. In the first case the maids may do a late shift e.g. 2–10 p.m. on a rota system or there may be evening maids separate from the morning ones who work the hours required e.g. 5–9 p.m. or 5–10 p.m. Some hotels cannot implement straight shifts and split duties may still be necessary. In these cases a maid may work 3 or 4 straight shifts and 1 or 2 split duties per week. (See p. 58.)

During the course of her work she may have half an hour for breakfast, and a mid-morning break of 15–20 minutes is taken in the staff canteen or her service room. Lunch will probably be 12–12.30 p.m. or 12.30–1 p.m. and at arranged times during the day according to house custom she will deal with soiled linen and replenish her cleaning stores and stock of clean linen.

Her first duty is to report to the duty housekeeper, collect her keys and relevant information regarding her section. Her last duty is putting in hot water bottles or switching on electric blankets where necessary, locking her cupboards and service room doors and handing in her keys to the duty housekeeper as she reports off duty.

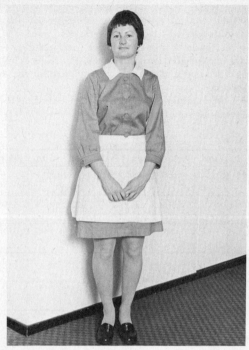

A room-maid's uniform

In some hotels maids live in; in others they live in a hostel or house provided for them, while in others they are non-resident, but in all cases they have their meals in the hotel either in the staff canteen or their service room when on duty. In the past it was customary for a room-maid to wear a print dress, a large white apron and mob cap in the mornings, and a dark dress, a head band and frilly apron in the evenings. Nowadays with the advent of easy care materials, overalls have replaced this uniform, and in some cases maids have to provide their own overalls and keep them laundered. Caps are not worn so frequently now, but maids are still required to wear stockings and sensible shoes.

There is little chance of promotion for a room-maid unless she moves to another hotel, as it would be unwise to make her an assistant housekeeper over those with whom she has been working on an equal footing.

In hotels coverage varies, e.g. 7 a.m.–9 p.m. or 8 a.m.–10 p.m. etc.; maids may work straight shifts or split duties and have 1½ or 2 days off per week.

In the example of a duty roster given, coverage is from 7 a.m.–4 p.m. and 5–10 p.m. except on Sundays; split duties have been included and the maids have one full day and two half days off per week. The roster is for 5 maids with no relief covering 5 sections and it might be advisable for the Sunday duties to rotate every 5 weeks.

46 hours is over the maximum number of hours according to the Catering Wages Order so overtime would have to be paid.

Maids	Mon.	Tues.	Wed.	Thurs.	Fri.	Sat.	Sun.	Wkly Hrs.
A	D.O.	8.30–2 6–10	7–2 5–9	8.30–2 6–10	7–2	7–4 (7–3.30)	7–2	46½ (46)
B	7–2	D.O.	8.30–2 6–10	7–4	7–2 5–9	7–4	3–10	46
C	7–4	7–2	D.O.	7–2 5–9	7–4	8.30–2 6–10	7–2	46
D	7–2 5–9	7–4	7–2	D.O.	8.30–2 6–10	7–4	2–9	46
E	8.30–2 6–10	7–2 5–9	7–4	7–2	D.O.	8.30–2 (8.30– 1.30) 5–9	7–2	46½ (46)

Mealtimes:

Breakfast   8–8.30 a.m. or 8.30–9.0 a.m.
Lunch   12–12.30 p.m. or 12.30–1 p.m.
Supper   6.30–7 p.m. or 7–7.30 p.m.

½ hr. allowed for tea on Sundays 4–4.30 p.m. or 4.30–5 p.m.

7–2	= 7 hrs. less 1 hr. = 6 hrs.
7–4	= 9 hrs. less 1 hr. = 8 hrs.
7–2 5–9	= 11 hrs. less 1½ hr. = 9½ (14 hrs. spread over)
8.30–2 5–9	= 9½ hrs. less 1 hr. = 8½ (12½ hrs. spread over)
8.30–2 6–10	= 9½ hrs. less 1 hr. = 8½ (13½ hrs. spread over)
2–9	= 7 hrs. less 1 hr. = 6 hrs.
3–10	= 7 hrs. less 1 hr. = 6 hrs.

AN ALTERNATIVE METHOD OF SETTING OUT THE SAME ROSTER.

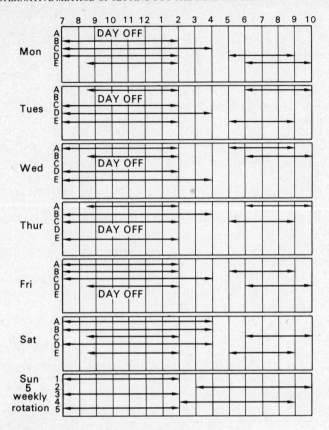

From the roster it can be assumed that:

1 The five maids are servicing approximately 60 rooms.
2 Maids will be serving early morning teas.
3 Guests require a certain amount of service in the evening.
4 Saturday is likely to be the day on which the greatest number of change overs take place.
5 On a day when a maid is off, the remaining four maids will service a split section in addition to their own.
6 A housekeeper will be available from 4–5 p.m. when there are no maids on duty.

The maid's hours could be cut by:

1 Floor waiters serving early morning teas or by the provision of 'do-it-yourself' equipment in the rooms.
2 Cutting down on the amount of night service
   a) one maid on instead of two.
   b) maids going off earlier in the evening (shorter coverage).

Staffmaids

In some hotels there is a staffmaid who services the rooms of assistant housekeepers and other living-in staff. If staffmaids look after maids' rooms they are more likely to report a lack of hygiene and in some cases 'livestock'. They usually work a straight shift, and may be part-time, and are considered when a room-maid's job falls vacant.

Cleaners

In the past, room-maids were assisted by housemaids, corridor or bathroom maids but today, owing to the shortage of staff, cleaners have replaced them. Cleaners are usually part-time, always live out, have their meals in the staff canteen when on duty, and usually they wear a coloured overall provided by the hotel. Their hours will vary according to the work they have to do; they may clean public rooms, ladies' cloakrooms, and offices before breakfast, and afterwards public bathrooms, toilets, corridors and stairs, and staff rooms where there is no staffmaid. Some hotels use contract cleaners (see p. 275).

(Cloakrooms for men are looked after by porters belonging to the uniform staff and in addition to the normal fittings and fixtures may contain urinals, usually of the stall type.)

Cloakroom attendant

In an hotel which has many functions and many non-resident guests, it is usual to have someone on duty during lunch and dinner periods in a ladies' powder room who attends to the requirements of the guests, guards their belongings and keeps the powder room neat and tidy. The initial cleaning of the powder room will have been done by a cleaner. If there is a need for the cloakroom attendant to be on duty in the powder room between 12–3 p.m. and again from 6–11 p.m. this will be a full-time job. Often, however, the powder room is cleaned by cleaners in the morning, checked several times during the day by an assistant housekeeper and only 'manned' when required. Thus, the cloakroom attendant may be part-time, or may be a linen room maid or a staff-maid, who does not normally work in the evenings and will take on this work as an extra. She wears either a dark dress and a frilly apron, or a white overall.

Houseporters

In the majority of hotels the houseporter is the only man on the house-keeping staff, and he may start work at 7 a.m. and does a straight day, working until 4 or 5 p.m. with appropriate meal breaks, taken in the staff canteen, working approximately a forty hour week.

The houseporter's duties will vary from one hotel to another, but as a rule, if there are coal fires to be dealt with, these will be his first job; on the other hand, he may help with the cleaning of the foyer and public rooms, do the heavier vacuum cleaning, the shaking of door mats, the cleaning of lamps and shades and possibly dusting large mirrors. He keeps the 'tools' for his work in a cupboard allotted to him.

After his breakfast half hour there will be certain jobs that he will carry out each day, and others only when requested, and circumstances will dictate if and when he does the following work:

replenishes cleaning stores according to house custom;
cleans brasses, e.g. stair rods and fire fighting equipment;
moves furniture, e.g. cots, bed boards;
spot cleans and maybe shampoos carpets;
takes linen to and from the floors;
empties rubbish;
helps maids with the moving of heavy furniture and the cleaning of
    high ledges and fitments;
takes down and rehangs curtains;
keeps fire buckets filled with sand or water;
carries coal.

The houseporter usually wears a denim or a buff coloured drill coat or jacket and apron provided by the hotel.

Valet-porters

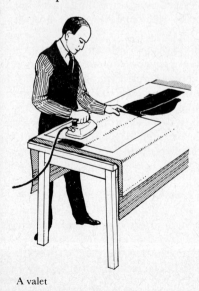

A valet

Valeting is only carried out on the premises of first class hotels and involves looking after the male guests, sponging, pressing and doing minor repairs to clothes, cleaning shoes, parcelling personal laundry, moving guests' belongings when changes of rooms are necessary, unpacking and packing for the guests. In the past a full-time valet was not on the housekeeping staff; he was either self-employed or on the uniform staff. However in newer hotels he may now be a member of the housekeeping staff because many of his duties e.g. moving guests' belongings, are the direct concern of the housekeeper.

In many instances a valet is not fully employed with valeting alone and so a valet-porter combines the work of a valet with the less dirty jobs of the houseporter and is a member of the housekeeping staff, so he may move furniture, transport linen, clean ledges and high lights, etc., but must retain his neat appearance as he is always on call to give personal service to guests.

The valet-porter has or shares a service room complete with iron and board, paper and string, needles and cotton, shoe cleaning necessities, and he usually keeps spare pyjamas, studs, braces, shoe laces, black ties, electric razors, etc., in case of emergencies.

A valet or valet-porter wears formal uniform trousers and an alpaca waistcoat with sleeves.

The assistant housekeeper

The main duties of the assistant housekeeper, floor housekeeper or floor supervisor are those concerned with the day to day running of the department, the supervision of the maids, cleaners and houseporters and the checking of rooms. The satisfaction of the guests with regard to the appearance and cleanliness of their rooms rests with the assistant housekeeper. In addition she may be given extra responsibilities by the housekeeper such as the issuing of cleaning stores or the keeping of lists for blanket and curtain changes etc. (see Chapter 1)

In all aspects of her work, she must be aware of company, 'house' and departmental policies and it is a help if she has had some period of induction before starting 'on the job'. No two hotels or housekeeping departments are run exactly alike so even a newly appointed assistant housekeeper with experience has things to learn concerning the work of a particular 'house'.

It has been suggested that there should be one assistant housekeeper for every 50 rooms but as the assistants are never all on duty at the same time due to rest days, shifts, etc., the actual number of rooms one assistant is responsible for in a large hotel may be nearer 100 or even more. Ideally the assistant housekeeper will make two visits to a vacated room; one before the maid enters the room, when lost property, missing or damaged articles and jobs required for maintenance will be noted, and the second when the maid has completed servicing the room and the assistant housekeeper checks it thoroughly prior to passing it to reception as a ready room (ready for letting).

In practice, because of the number of rooms, the assistant housekeeper often has to rely on the maid reporting promptly any lost property, missing or damaged articles etc. she finds in the room. The assistant housekeeper not only makes sure that her maids understand about these things but also about the need for fire precautions, the care of keys, the way of dealing with strangers on the floors as well as other aspects of safety and security.

The assistant housekeeper should be friendly towards her maids without undue familiarity, firm, fair, constructively critical and should give praise where praise is due.

During the course of her work the assistant housekeeper has to be observant, quick and thorough. She carries a master key which opens all bedroom doors and she may be dismissed should she lose this key, she also carries a clipboard and pencil. As she goes round her floor she makes notes regarding her visits to the rooms and details such items as light luggage, extra departures, packed luggage, extra furniture, jobs for maintenance etc. At any time she may have interruptions from guests making requests or complaints, and from maids wanting advice and also there will be cleaners and houseporters to deal with.

It is usual to have a housekeeper's office where the housekeeper may discuss the affairs of the day with her assistants and to which they may return from time to time to enter details in the diary, maintenance book etc., and to receive information regarding extra departures, late departures, moves etc. and where they may sit to do necessary paper work.

The first job of the assistant housekeeper on early morning duty will be to check in the maids and cleaners, issue keys, early call and morning tea lists and other relevant information and at night the last duty will be to check the return of all keys and lock them away according to house custom (see p. 269).

In large hotels where there will be a number of assistant housekeepers (floor housekeepers or floor supervisors) it is usual for there to be a senior assistant, first assistant or deputy head (or executive) housekeeper who will act for the head housekeeper in her absence. The senior assistant housekeeper may undertake the checking of some rooms, particularly rooms for VIPs, and rooms out of order. She is normally responsible for the day to day running of the department, the allocation of staff, the compiling of duty rosters and holiday lists, and the keeping of staff records including hours worked by staff for wage calculations.

In hotels where there is a housekeeper with only one or two assistants an assistant housekeeper may be on duty alone and will deputise for the housekeeper when necessary and is sometimes called the duty housekeeper. In such hotels, the housekeeper herself may at times be the only one on duty and is therefore much more involved in the day to day routine of the checking of rooms etc. than the head or executive housekeeper in a large hotel.

In many small hotels there are no assistant housekeepers and a general assistant will combine housekeeping with many other duties e.g. reception and the bar.

The hours of work for an assistant housekeeper will vary tremendously. There will be hotels where assistants work straight shifts such as 8 hours a day 5 days a week e.g. 7 a.m.–3 p.m., 9 a.m.–5 p.m., 2 p.m.–10 p.m., 3 p.m.–11 p.m. or they may have to work some split duties e.g. 8 a.m.–2 p.m., 6 p.m.–10 p.m. so that the necessary hours of coverage for the department are met. In hotels where a 24 hour coverage is needed for the housekeeping department there may be a night housekeeper who could work for example 11 p.m.–7 a.m. Minimum wages and holidays, and maximum working hours are laid down by the Catering Wages Regulation Order. The assistant may be resident or non-resident and takes her meals in the steward's room though in newer hotels there may be a canteen where all staff feed. In some hotels assistant housekeepers wear a black dress of their own choice while in others they may wear a uniform provided by the hotels.

The aim of the assistant is to become a housekeeper and any further qualifications that she can acquire such as a foreign language or HCITB certificates (e.g. Instructor trainers' course) will be a help in her present work and towards her promotion.

Suggested method of procedure by an assistant housekeeper when checking a bedroom with a private bathroom for a new arrival

1   In a clockwise or anti-clockwise direction check systematically everything on or touching the walls:
e.g.   electric light switches, telephone, radio and television;
  bed—making up, clean linen, castors, headboard, etc., bed light, bedside cabinet and contents;
  dressing table—clean and re-lined drawers, drawer stops, mirror, disclaimer notice, laundry lists, etc.;
  wardrobe—clean shelves, rail, coat hangers, mirror, hinge and lock of door;
  window—sill, sashcords, catches, curtains, pelmet and runners;
  radiators;
  luggage rack;
  picture;
  door—top, architrave and lock.

2   Check free standing furniture:
e.g.   armchair—upholstery, chair back, castors;
  occasional table and ashtrays;
  dressing table stool;
  waste-paper basket.

3   Check ceiling and floor:
e.g.   cobwebs;
  central lights;
  floor—carpet, surround, etc.

4   General surveyance of the room.
5   Private Bathroom
e.g.   light switch;

Vanitory unit—mirror, tiles, toothglass, light, razor point, taps, basin (underside, overflow, plug and waste hole), new soap, clean towels and guests' supplies;

W.C.—bowl inside and out, underside of seat and lid, toilet paper;

Ashtray and sanibin;

Bath and shower—tiles, chrome fittings, soap recesses, the tub (overflow, plug and waste hole), towel rack, shower curtain and rail, new soap, bath mat and non slip rubber mat according to house custom;

Door—top, architrave, lock and hook;

Ceiling and floor;

General surveyance of room.

N.B. This is assuming the bathroom is internal; should there be a window then sill, catches, curtains and runners should be checked. In more luxury hotels there may be a bidet which would be checked in a similar manner to the W.C.

Any other items in the room not already mentioned should be dealt with systematically, and all maintenance work, and discrepancies found in the maids' work, should be written down and dealt with accordingly.

Staff Duties in Non-Commercial Establishments

As in most establishments other than hotels, the staffing is for cleaning and there is little personal service, the hours worked by the cleaners will depend on the areas to be maintained by the housekeeping department and the number of staff employed to undertake that work. As many of the staff will be part-time cleaners their hours will determine the amount of work which can be assigned to each employee.

In various types of hostels little work can be done before 9 a.m. so cleaners may work from 9 a.m.–1 p.m., 9 a.m.–3 p.m. or even 9.30 a.m.–3.30 p.m. and so the amount of work assigned to them will vary. The *housekeepers* will man the department at other times as the department requires. There are hostels and 'homes' where cleaners start earlier, e.g. 6.45 or 7 a.m., and this may be the case where public rooms are required to be cleaned before breakfast, in nurses' homes where sisters may be called at 7 a.m. and night nurses' rooms have to be cleaned before the nurses come off duty. A cleaner may also be required for a few hours in the evening, e.g. 5.30–7.30 p.m. in the nurses' home for the calling of night sisters and the taking of meals to sick nurses, etc.

In any of these residential establishments cleaners are hindered by residents being in their rooms and it is generally recognised that there will be days when the very minimum amount of work will be done in a particular room due to it being occupied. In students' hostels this applies especially at weekends and in many cases there will be no cleaners in on Saturday or Sunday for the cleaning of the study bedrooms. Occasionally there may be a few full-time maids—possibly resident—whose duty rosters will be arranged so that they may clean public rooms, vacated guest rooms where these are provided, and similar jobs which become necessary. Thorough cleaning of students' hostels is normally carried out each vacation when the rooms are empty but difficulties do arise, as for the economic running of the hostels facilities have to be available for conferences during the major part of the vacations. Careful planning should be given to the letting of the hostels for such conferences to enable the extra cleaning including annual cleaning with possible redecoration to be carried out. In other establishments thorough and annual cleaning will be carried on throughout the year as is convenient to the particular place.

Cleaners in some establishments are required to clock in and where the establishment is large this presents problems as there is an inevitable time lag between clocking in, getting their keys and getting to their place of work.

Cleaners

Cleaners in various types of hostels and halls of residence may service a section of 10–20 rooms with or without wash basins, utility room, bathrooms, W.C.'s, showers and corridor. Assuming the cleaner starts work at approximately 9 a.m. she will probably clean the rooms of her section either completing each in one visit or doing one job throughout a number of rooms and so on until the work is completed.

In many instances the beds will be made by the residents and the cleaners will only make them on clean sheet day. As probably no cleaning is done at the weekends, the rooms on Mondays will need a little more attention and so Mondays should be avoided as the day when the linen is changed. It is usual to send the bottom sheet and one pillowslip to the laundry each week and so the top sheet becomes the bottom sheet and a clean one is put on the top. Thus one clean sheet and one clean pillowslip are provided each week. (The residents often provide their own towels.)

A mid-morning break of about 15 minutes is usual and it is possible that about this time on given days the cleaner will collect her cleaning stores according to house custom. If the cleaner works after 1 p.m. she will be given ½–1 hour break for lunch which she will probably take between 12 noon and 2 p.m. After her lunch she continues her work and before going off duty deals with her equipment and hands in her key.

If there are areas, e.g. offices, which require cleaning before breakfast they will either be dealt with by a living-in maid or a cleaner who comes in early. Other areas, e.g. entrance halls, common rooms, dining rooms, etc., will be cleaned at a time convenient to the house.

The daily routine for cleaners in places let during vacations for conferences, summer schools, etc., may be considerably different from that during term time. The guests may require more service e.g. bed making and rooms may be let for comparatively short periods so there may be very little time for cleaning between one let and the next. The cleaners normally have a share of the block tips.

It is usual for a cleaner to wear an overall which may or may not be provided by the establishment.

Male domestics (porters)

Male domestics (porters) in various types of hostels and halls of residence can be likened to houseporters in an hotel and their duties may include dealing with rubbish, moving of furniture, cleaning carpets, cleaning fire escapes, transporting linen, etc. They may wear a denim coat or dungarees and will work such hours as are required by the establishment.

Forewomen/supervisors

In large establishments where there are many cleaners and large areas to cover, there may be forewomen/supervisors who are responsible for the day-to-day control of a number of cleaners in a particular area.

Assistant housekeepers/junior domestic bursars

The main work of an assistant housekeeper is the supervision of the cleaners and the checking of the rooms. During this time she makes out maintenance lists according to house custom and checks that previous maintenance work has been carried out. Any urgent repairs will be immediately reported to the appropriate person. In addition to the above work she fits in any work delegated to her by the housekeeper/domestic bursar.

One assistant housekeeper will be on duty just before the cleaners start work to check them in, issue keys, pass on information and rearrange the work of absentees. Assistant housekeepers will normally work some split shifts as it is usual to have one of them on call in the evening.

Until recent years the *Domestic Services of Hospitals* have been the responsibility of the Nursing Administration. With the coming realisation that nurses are trained to nurse and should not spend valuable time on work that does not require nurse training, these duties have now become the prerogative of lay staff trained in Domestic Management. This encompasses all the new developments in up-to-date cleaning equipment and techniques required for the proper cleaning of hospital premises and other duties that do not require nursing skills—e.g. serving of food, linen services etc. In 1968 a sub-committee of the Standing Nursing Advisory Committee published its findings in a report 'Relieving Nurses of Non-Nursing Duties in General and Maternity Hospitals'. The Committee recommended a new non-nursing staffing pattern based on housekeeping teams being introduced into wards to replace all grades of non-nursing staff now employed on wards.

The domestic superintendent/manager is responsible for the housekeeping of all parts of the hospital including staff residences.

This involves vast floor areas which are in use twenty-four hours a day and three hundred and sixty-five days a year. Special areas such as intensive care unit, theatres, renal unit, transplant unit and premature baby unit are also included and accurate planning of work schedules is necessary, for the availability of these areas is limited, and they often have to be cleaned outside normal hours.

Domestic Assistants, Ward Orderlies and Room Cleaners

The above grades are employed to relieve nurses of non-nursing duties on patient areas and to clean all other parts of the hospital. Many domestic staff now work under incentive bonus scheme conditions.

Domestic Supervisors/Ward Housekeepers

The supervisors or ward housekeepers are first line managers who supervise the work of the domestic assistants and ward orderlies in a given area and are responsible to the domestic superintendent for maintaining the correct methods of work and standards. They are responsible for the training and allocation of staff in their areas to ensure that the correct methods and standards are maintained. They liaise with the ward sisters/charge nurses on the work within the wards.

Assistant Domestic Superintendents and Senior Housekeepers

Depending on the size of the hospital a domestic superintendent is supported by a number of assistant domestic superintendents or senior housekeepers. When a hospital is too small to justify the appointment of a domestic superintendent an assistant domestic superintendent or senior housekeeper will be responsible to the District Domestic Services Manager or Hospital Secretary for the supervision of domestic services.

Date

WARD/DEPARTMENT	STANDARD			Action taken by Supervisor
	Good	Fair	Poor	
Carpets				
Vacuum cleaned				
Spot free				
Floors				
Vacuum cleaned				
Damp mopped				
Dressed and buffed				
Furniture and fittings				
Damp mopped				
Polished				
Upholstery vacuumed				
Sinks, basin				
Spot free				
Inside				
Outside				
Underneath				
Taps				
Plughole, plug, and chain				
Overflow and fitments				
Lavatories				
Inside				
Outside				
Underneath				
Backs				
Seat				
Chain				
Brush holder				
Baths				
Inside				
Outside				
Underneath				
Taps				
Plughole, plug and chain				
Overflow and fitments				
High cleaning				
Curtain rails				
Door ledges				
Tops of cupboards				
Ledges, pipes				
Low cleaning				
Corners				
Pipes				
Radiators				
Wheels				
Under furniture				
Rubbish				
Ashtrays				
Disposal bags and stands				
Incinerators				

Specimen checklist. (Hospitals).

LOST PROPERTY

DATE FOUND: ....
WHERE FOUND: ....
FINDERS NAME: .... Dept: ....

DESCRIPTION OF ARTICLE:

FOR OFFICE USE

REGISTER ENTRY No. ....
DATE .... INITIALS ....
DISPOSAL: ....

Chambermaids Occupancy Report

Date: ....

Room No.	Vacant or Occupied	No. Sleepers	Room No.	Vacant or Occupied	No. Sleepers
501			509		
502			510		
503			511		
504			512		
505			514		
506			515		
507			516		
508			517		

To be handed in to the Housekeeper Office each morning by 10.30 a.m.

Signature: ....

HOUSEKEEPERS ROOM REPORT

LIGHT BAGGAGE. Write L.B., in Remarks Column when room contains only light baggage.

Time: ....
Date: .... 19....
Floor No.: ....
Inspection by: ....

Room No.	Does Lock? Yes/No	Does'nt Reg'tr Yes/No	Bath in Room	Not Slept in	Vacant	Out of Order	REMARKS
1							
2							
3							
4							
5							
6							
7							
8							
9							
10							
11							
12							
13							
14							
15							
16							
17							
18							
19							
20							
21							
22							
23							

FLOOR SHEET

FLOOR ....   DATE ....
                        TIME ....

No.	OCC	VAC	COMMENTS	No.	OCC	VAC	COMMENTS
01				21			
02				22			
03				23			
04				24			
05				25			
06				26			
07				27			
08				28			
09				29			
10				30			
11				31			
12				32			
14				33			
15				34			
16				35			
17				36			
18				37			
19							
20							

H/K signature ....

Reception signature ....

INN ON THE PARK

DATE: ....   TIME: ....

6th FLOOR

FLOOR CHECKING SHEETS

ROOM No.	LET	VAC.	No. of Persons	Cot or E.B.		
601						
602						
603						
604						
605						
606						
607						
608						
609						
610						
611						
612						
613						
614						
616						
618						
619						
620						
621						
622						
623						
624						
625						
626						
627						
628						
629						
630						
632						

Signature ....

A22866

Specimen record sheets (Hotels).

ROOM NO.	STATUS	ROOM NO.	STATUS	ROOM NO.	STATUS	ROOM NO.	STATUS
01	OCC	19	OCC	E.D. 36	OCC	53	OCC
02	OCC	20	CR	37	Vac	54	
03	CR	21	OCC	38	OCC	55	
04	OCC	22	OCC	39	OCC	56	
05	Vac	23	OOO	40	CR	58	
06	OCC	24	OCC	41	CR	HAND-OVER	
07	OCC	25	OCC	42	CR	509 -Table Light	
08	CR	26	OCC	43	CR	517- Lobby Light OOO	
09	CR	27	N.G.	44	OCC	514- Not packed	
10	OCC	28	CR	45	Vac	505 Late service	
11	OCC	29	OCC	46	OCC	518 Not packed	
12	OCC	30	OCC	47	OCC		
14	N.P.	31	OCC	48	N.P.		
15	CR	32	OCC	49	OCC		
16	CR	33	CR	50	OCC		
17	OCC	34	CR	51	OCC		
18	OCC	35	OCC	52	OCC		

CR = checked and ready   ED = Extra departure
NP = Not packed   OOO = out of order
NG = Not going

Signature _P.J.Webb._

Specimen floor check list (Hotels).

GENERAL MAINTENANCE REPORT

Dept: Housekeeping   Floor _5th_   Signature _Sue Woolt_   Date _29-3-74_

ITEM	ROOM NUMBER								
CONSTRUCTION									
Bedroom curtains—a) track b) runners									
Bath—a) tap b) slow waste c) plug off d) stained	501ᵃ								
e) chipped f) seal									
Basin—a) tap b) slow waste c) plug off d) stained									
e) cracked f) seal									
Bathroom flooring —a) marked b) torn c) loose	584ᵃ	523ᵃ	511ᶜ						
Chairs—a) broken b) dirty c) torn									
Carpet—a) minor repair b) spot c) shampoo	503ᵇ								
Dressing table drawers—a) broken b) handles off									
Dado rail—a) off b) torn									
Door closer—a) not working properly									
Furniture—a) cigarette burns									
Loose/defective fittings—a) hooks b) towel rail									
c) door stops d) bottle openers e) drip dries	571ᶜ	588ᴰ							
f) tissue dispenser									
Mirror—a) cracked b) spotted c) domeheads	564ᵃ								
Paintwork—a) chipped b) dirty									
Polishing—a) door b) furniture									
Shower curtain —a) track b) runners									
Threshold strip to bathroom —a) loose b) off									
Toilet seat— a) loose b) chipped									
Wall tiles—a) cracked									
W.C.—a) stained b) cracked									
Wardrobe—a) catches b) shelf c) hinges d) hanging									
rail									
Window—a) not opening b) not closing c) not									
CORRIDORS fastening									
Ceiling sections—a) missing b) dirty									
Signs—a) loose b) broken c) missing									
Wall covering—a) torn b) dirty									
ELECTRICIANS									
Bedhead console switches—a) knobs loose									
b) missing									
Bathroom extract—a) dirty b) not working									
Lobby light—a) not working									
Lampshades—a) chipped b) cracked									
Room status indicator—a) not working									
ENGINEERS									
Extract —a) dirty									
Room 529 Double lock not working									

BATHROOM INSPECTION REPORT

Ashtrays	
Bottle Opener	
Bath exterior	
Bath interior	
Bath overflow	
Bath plug chain	
Bath shower	
Bath taps	
Bath wastes	
Bath hand grip	
Non-slip mat	
Basin interior	
Basin overflow	
Basin plug chain	
Basin surround	
Basin taps	
Basin tumblers	
Door tops	
Door jambs	
Floors	
Light	
Mirror	
Razor envelopes	
Sanitary bags	
Shower caps	
Soap holders	
Stocking rail	
Toilet cistern	
Toilet exterior	
Toilet interior	
Toilet seat top	
Toilet under	
Toilet lid	
Roll holder space	
Tissue box	
Tiles	
Towel rails	
Ventilator	
Wastepaper bin	

Housekeeper's signature......................   Room nos Inspected..............

BEDROOM INSPECTION REPORT

Miss Johnson

	581 VAC	571 VAC	574 OCC	583 DEP
Ashtrays	✓	✓	✓	✓
Bed making	✓		✓	✓
Bed wheels	✓	dusty	✓	✓
Bed head	✓		✓	✓
Bed sides	slight dust	✓	✓	✓
Bed unit	✓	✓	✓	✓
Blotter contents	✓	stained	✓	✓
Carpets	not hoovered	✓	not hoovered	✓
Carpet edges	neglected	neglected	✓	neglected
Chair arms		✓	✓	
Chair dressing table	✓	✓	✓	✓
Coat hangers	✓	✓	✓	not enough supplied
Dressing table unit	✓	✓	✓	
Drawers	✓	✓	✓	not checked
Door tops	✓	✓	✓	
Door Comm.	✓	✓	✓	✓
Door jambs	✓	✓	✓	✓
Furniture	✓	✓	✓	✓
Furniture fronts	✓	✓	✓	✓
Furniture legs	✓	✓	✓	✓
Lobby skirting	✓	✓	✓	✓
Lobby carpet	not hoovered	not hoovered	not hoovered	not hoovered
Lights bedside	✓	✓		
Lights dressing table	✓	slight dust	✓	✓
Lights standard lamp	✓		✓	✓
Laundry bags (2)	✓	✓	✓	only 1
Mirrors	✓	✓	✓	
Pictures	✓	✓	top of picture dusty	✓
Skirtings	✓	✓		✓
Tables Coffee	stained	✓	✓	✓
Tables bedside	✓	✓	✓	✓
Telephones	✓	✓	✓	✓
Ventilator	✓	✓	✓	✓
Wardrobe shelves	✓	✓	✓	good
Wardrobe floor	✓	✓	✓	✓
Wardrobe rack	✓	✓	✓	✓
Wardrobe rail	✓	✓	✓	✓
Window ledges	✓	✓	✓	good
Wastepaper bin	✓	ash still in bin	✓	✓

Housekeeper's signature A.J.Wilson ....

3

The Linen Room

The linen room is the central depot for all linen and from it sufficient clean articles, in good condition, are distributed throughout the house.

Linen, in this context, means launderable articles, but the linen room staff may also handle blankets, curtains, loose covers as well as articles for dry cleaning.

(N.B. 'Linen' is the only fibre name which also applies to a fabric. Cotton, nylon, terylene, etc., are fibre names and the fabrics made from them may be, for example, cotton sheeting, cotton damask, nylon damask, nylon brocade, terylene net, etc., or in general terms cotton fabrics, nylon fabrics, etc.)

When one considers that even for a small establishment many hundreds of articles are necessary for the bedrooms alone, it will be realised that the linen keeper (under the supervision of the *housekeeper*) has a great responsibility for the control of this stock.

There will be establishments where a great deal of linen is handled, e.g. in hospitals, or in hotels where there is much banqueting and daily re-sheeting. In these places there may be a linen keeper with several assistants. In small establishments where less linen is handled the work may be done by the general assistant or a linen maid.

In hostels for various types of people and similar places where complete re-sheeting for the residents is usually once a fortnight (i.e. one sheet, one pillowslip per week and residents may provide their own towels) very much less linen is handled and so a linen maid may do the work part-time.

The linen keeper or person in charge of the linen room, except in hospitals, is responsible according to house custom for the issue of all linen, the sorting and despatch of the soiled linen to the laundry, the checking on its return and for its general standard. According to house custom she keeps as strict a control as possible over the exchange of soiled for clean linen. She should be able to be firm with the laundry manager over such difficulties as careless laundering and losses, and she should keep the record books accurately and efficiently.

Linen room work in hotels

The hours that the linen room is open will vary: 8 a.m.–5 p.m. for a large hotel is usual, but in other cases there may be a set time, possibly twice a day, always remembering that the linen room is normally open seven days a week. When closed, the door should always be locked and the key taken to the reception or the housekeeper's office according to the custom of the house.

Uniform for the linen room staff consists of white overalls provided by the hotel and laundered free. A head linen keeper has her meals in the couriers' or stewards' room and the assistants have theirs in the staff hall, but in new hotels, there may be a staff canteen for all grades of staff.

In the event of linen being required during the night, the duty manager or night porter may have his own small store, or he may remove items from the linen room and leave a note with details of what has been removed. No unauthorised persons are allowed access to the linen room.

The rule of 'clean for dirty' is considered the best way of keeping control on linen with regard to losses and careless use, and the most usual ways of exchanging linen are:

(*a*) directly over the counter by the maid, waiter, plongeur, cleaner, house and kitchen porters.
(*b*) the listed and bundled soiled linen is taken to the linen room by the maid, house or linen porter at a set time each day and the clean linen is later collected or returned.
(*c*) the soiled linen is despatched down a linen chute and the floor stock of clean linen is made up later in the day by the house or linen porter.

In a large hotel it is not practical for a maid to make several journeys to the linen room to exchange her soiled linen directly over the counter so she has a supply of linen in reserve, usually enough to resheet her section and this reserve is kept in a floor linen cupboard under lock and key and is made up each day after the soiled linen has been sent to the linen room. While with the chute there is not the same check possible there is great saving of time.

It is important that soiled linen should be sent to the linen room as soon as possible for despatch to the laundry, since if it is left lying about, misuse is more frequent, and if in a damp condition, iron mould and mildew can occur, and both these stains need special treatment for their removal. Badly stained articles should be sent to the laundry separately from other soiled linen, so that they may receive special attention, which is an added expense.

As far as possible, similar items are placed in one basket, and care must be taken that no tapes or corners are left hanging out as they may get torn or badly marked. Linen is usually transported in wicker baskets (size approximately 75 cm x 45 cm) firmly fastened by straps, but sometimes canvas bags or vinyl hampers are used. With the soiled linen, a list of all items sent to the laundry is given to the vanman and the duplicate copy is kept in the linen room. It is necessary to keep the baskets with soiled linen apart from those with clean, as mistakes can easily be made.

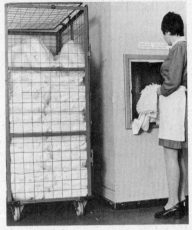

A linen chute

As soon as possible after the vanman has delivered the clean linen, the baskets are opened and the articles counted on to the inspection table. 'Shorts' are noted and entered on the next day's laundry list. In some large hotels the laundry sends a checker to count with one of the linen room maids, the soiled linen going to and the clean linen returning from the laundry. In this way time is saved and there is less likelihood of misunderstandings arising over numbers of articles sent to and returned from the laundry. Ideally, after counting the clean linen and before it is put on the shelves, it should be inspected for:

    repairs,
    stains,
    very bad creasing,
    articles belonging to other hotels.

This means that each article has to be opened out and, if necessary, put aside for mending or for return to the laundry for exchange or re-wash. Badly torn articles or 'light' linen, i.e. linen worn thin, are put on one side for the housekeeper or linen keeper to condemn or discard, to enter in the 'condemned' book and later to mark off in the stock book.

Skilled workers can inspect large articles alone by holding them up to the light, or by placing them flat on the table, but it is often quicker if two linen maids work together, and when inspecting large numbers of small articles, e.g. napkins, it is less tiring if the maids are provided with chairs.

If inspection is carried out thoroughly on all articles, always providing there is sufficient staff, it means a high standard of linen is maintained, and the chance of a guest having a napkin with a stain on it or a sheet with a hole in it is less likely, and the linen has a longer life owing to a 'stitch in time saving nine'. Work study experts have observed that in some situations the 'inspection' of the linen could be omitted. They suggest that it could be made the responsibility of the users, e.g. waiters and room-maids; however, housekeepers and linen keepers who take a pride in their linen, argue that if inspection is omitted, then standards must be lowered because careless workers will either use the damaged article, or put it with the soiled linen so that it goes to the laundry again, and room-maids will waste much time when there is no floor linen stock, in going to exchange faulty articles. Time and labour may be saved in the linen room by the laundry returning the linen in packs, a single pack consisting of 2 sheets, 2 pillowslips and towels according to house custom. In this way counting packs is easier than counting individual articles and inspection is cut in the linen room.

Where a laundry operates on the premises, the inspection could be the responsibility of the laundry workers, and linen for repair could then be kept separate and sent direct to the repair department.

However, each situation must be considered on its own merits, and linen standards must be balanced against savings in time and wages. There are hotels which hire their linen instead of buying it and in these cases the amount of work in the linen room will be less because of less stock, no inspection and no repairs. As a result of this less staff is needed.

In an hotel it is usual to put a laundry list and sometimes a container, such as a large paper bag, as well as a dry cleaning list in all bedrooms for the guests' personal laundry. The guest is asked to complete the list, and to fill in the service required, e.g. normal or 'express', and the room-maid or valet takes the parcel to the linen room. The linen keeper enters the particulars into a guest laundry or dry cleaning book and the vanman collects the parcels.

On its return, the parcel is sent to the guest's room via the valet, room-maid or hall porter according to the custom of the house, and the amount to be charged on the guest's bill is given to the bill office. In some cases dry cleaning is not sent via the linen room but via the valet or hall porter.

Articles such as waiters' jackets, aprons, cleaners' overalls, are treated as normal linen stock, and exchanged over the counter, but, where the staff is provided with individual uniform, this is treated as personal laundry, and may be sent as individual bundles to the laundry and returned a week later. There are certain members of staff (amongst whom may be the assistant housekeepers) who have their 'dress' dry cleaned periodically at the hotel's expense and in a large hotel there may be a section of the linen room given over to the care of uniforms.

Linen room work in establishments other than hotels

While many of the already mentioned points concerning the work in

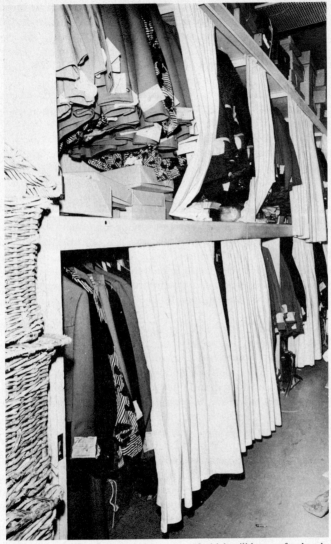

A section of the linen room for uniforms many of which will be sent for dry cleaning

the linen room may apply to establishments other than hotels, there are some important differences.

In hospitals, soiled linen is sent direct to the laundry from the individual places, wards, nurses' homes, etc. and infected and foul linen is always dealt with separately. In the past articles were marked with the name of the ward, etc., and the clean articles were returned direct to the ward etc. from the laundry and the linen room staff were mainly concerned with sewing. However, more usually now the articles are not individually marked, thus no sorting is necessary and the clean articles are returned to the wards, etc., via a central linen room. In either case there must be adequate storage space for the linen in the wards, nurses' homes, etc.

It is more hygienic when nurses send their soiled aprons to the laundry direct from the ward rather than taking them back to their rooms to be kept until the weekly collection day.

From the above it will be realised that in a hospital the rule of 'clean for dirty' is not normally applied and that it is more often a 'topping up' system, and inspection is kept to a minimum. Some hospitals are fortunate in that they require fewer paid sewing maids as help is given by voluntary workers.

In most hostels, collection and delivery of laundry will be weekly owing to the less frequent changing of linen. Consequently, unless there is much sewing dealt with in the linen room it need not be open every day. In many instances the rule of clean for dirty will not apply as the cleaners will be issued with clean linen before stripping the beds. Where the residents change their own beds they are sometimes expected to strip the bed and leave the soiled linen for the cleaners to pick up before the clean is left.

In all establishments, due to the high cost of labour, little hand sewing is done in a **linen room**, but a great deal of machining, and thus a sewing machine gets much use and needs to be kept in perfect order. Machines should be dusted and oiled by the operators, and an arrangement should be made for the regular servicing of them on contract. Good light for machining is essential as well as the necessary tools and equipment, such as needles, scissors and cotton.

For economy, mending should be carried out before laundering, but dealing with soiled and perhaps wet articles is not pleasant, so mending is usually done on clean linen. Any article not quite up to standard for guests' use in an hotel may be marked for staff or renovated and the last use of all linen is for rag which will be used for many cleaning purposes.

Straight-forward ordinary machining is used for hems on sheets or towels, patching, repairs to flaps of pillowslips, torn pockets, etc. In addition to these repairs, in some linen rooms the assistants make up new curtains, bedspreads, aprons, etc. When past repair, articles that are condemned may be economically used in the following ways:

1   Sheets made into under pillowslips, cot sheets, draw sheets, ironing board covers or used as linen covers and dust sheets.
2   Turkish and huckaback towels made into lavatory towels.

3 Table cloths made into sideboard and tray cloths.

4 Napkins used as chefs' neckties.

5 Thin bedspreads used for dust sheets.

6 Blankets used for under blankets, cot blankets and for padding ironing boards.

Thin places, small holes and cuts frequently occur in towels, table and bed linen, and these are repaired by machine darning. For this work it is necessary for the operator to use both hands, so an electrically powered or treadle machine is essential.

Machine marking may be carried out in the linen room and when marking linen it is usual to mark on the right side of the article, the name of the house or department and the date; the date is to show the age of the article and to check on its wearing quality.

This marking may be done on any linen except perhaps waiters' jackets, aprons, kitchen cloths, dusters, etc., which are more usually stamped.

The shelves on which the linen is stored should be firmly fixed, as the weight on them may be considerable, particularly the weight of large linen table cloths and sheets, and the shelves should be clearly marked for each type of article. They should reach to the ceiling and there should be room to mop or vacuum clean under the bottom shelf. In order that the linen should be kept aired, the room should be warm, and the shelves slatted to allow free circulation of air.

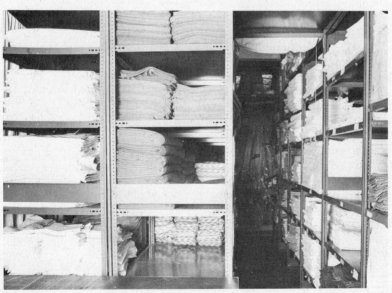

A linen room

During storage, linen must be kept free from dust, but it is inevitable that where linen is being handled, dust and fluff will occur and so all linen should be covered. Linen in constant use, may be covered by curtains which draw across the shelves, or stored in cupboards with sliding doors. In the case of less frequently used articles, e.g. special banqueting cloths, curtains and extra blankets, linen covers (often condemned sheets) may be used to wrap round them.

Linen wears better and lasts longer, if it is allowed to rest, and so a good stock of linen should be kept and always used in rotation. In order that there shall be rotation, all freshly laundered articles are put at the bottom or back of the pile. To make counting easier, linen is stacked with the folds outwards and small articles, e.g. napkins, are placed in tens, often nine, with the tenth wrapped round or secured with a rubber band.

As well as the storage of linen in normal use, a reserve stock needs to be kept, and this is frequently stored in its original packing paper after it has been checked, in a cupboard under lock and key. The cupboard may or may not be in the actual linen room, and there must be a list kept of this stock.

Many articles may be issued new and unlaundered, but tea towels and glass cloths are always laundered before issue, and a good linen keeper will have some of these stored ready laundered.

Launderable linen is required throughout the establishment, and thus the linen room is an essential and important place, and much thought should be given to its situation and planning in order that the work of issue, collection, storage and upkeep of the articles can go on as smoothly as possible.

Ideally, the linen room should be situated with direct and easy access for the loading and unloading of linen baskets to and from the laundry, and for the distribution of linen throughout the establishment.

In order that the work should be carried out efficiently the linen room should:

1   Be large enough for the necessary work to be carried on without overcrowding.

2   Have an easily cleaned floor which will withstand the dragging of baskets and which will not be too noisy or cold.

3   Have walls and ceiling of a light-coloured washable paint.

4   Have windows, if possible; in any case, lighting should be good and free from glare since many of the articles to be dealt with are white.

5   Have adequate ventilation and heating to prevent mildew forming on the stored linen and to keep it well aired.

6   Have slatted wooden shelves to allow free circulation of air.

7   Have a counter or stable type door over which articles may be exchanged, and to prevent the entry of unauthorised people.

8 Have a door with a strong lock for security reasons and wide enough to take laundry baskets and trolleys.

9 Have a wash basin, soap and towel.

In order to carry out this work, the staff will require:

(*a*) baskets or bags in which to pack soiled linen,
(*b*) a table as a working surface, of a colour to contrast with the white linen,
(*c*) a trolley or floor basket on wheels to save labour,
(*d*) steps to reach high shelves,
(*e*) sewing machines for repairing and marking the linen,
(*f*) an electric iron and ironing board or table,
(*g*) a suitable table or desk, with drawers for the keeping of record books,
(*h*) a telephone,
(*i*) chairs for those who may work seated,
(*j*) a broom, brush and dust pan or preferably a mop sweeper or vacuum cleaner.

Soiled linen on arrival at the linen room is sorted into bins. To prevent any confusion between soiled and clean linen baskets, the laundry man delivers the clean ones to I and picks up the soiled ones from J. See diagram overleaf.

From this diagram it will be seen that the principles of work study have been followed as far as possible.

Stocktaking is done at specified intervals in order to check the amount of linen, to know when to order new, and, if possible, to check the losses. It is frequently done monthly or three monthly, and in order to prevent discrepancies it is better if all stock is taken on the same day.

Every piece of linen throughout the establishment should be counted, and the number at the laundry according to the laundry book added. Stock is taken by responsible people in each department on the same day, and the lists handed in to the linen keeper who makes up the stock book.

Each page in the stock book will show the alterations in the linen stock for that particular stocktaking period, and when there are serious losses, the matter should be investigated and control tightened.

Although articles in the linen room have been described as launderable, it should be remembered that very much more use is being made of plastic and disposable materials which replace linen. Great advances have been made in the manufacture of plastic tablecloths, mats and traycloths. These are durable, economical in price and are not sent to

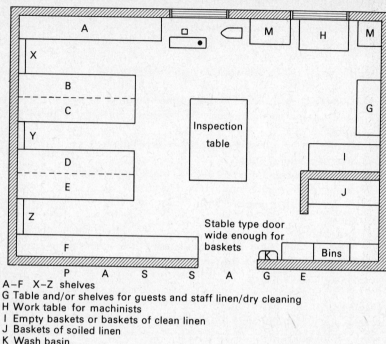

A–F X–Z shelves
G Table and/or shelves for guests and staff linen/dry cleaning
H Work table for machinists
I Empty baskets or baskets of clean linen
J Baskets of soiled linen
K Wash basin
M Machine

A suggested plan of a linen room.

the laundry; when soiled they are sponged or washed on the premises and they do not require mending.

Disposable articles are generally those thought of as being used once and then thrown away, e.g. paper napkins, tissues and hand towels, and from this point of view they are very hygienic.

There are 'disposables' made of rayon which may be used more than once and yet have a short life compared with their normal counterpart, e.g. bedlinen and cleaning cloths. In the case of bedlinen the articles may stand up to several nights use and are then thrown away; whereas the cleaning cloths depending on use and user, may be used once or may withstand several washings and further use.

These articles are hygienic, labour saving, disposable or short life but problems which must be overcome are the collection and disposal of the soiled articles and storage space for the new stock.

Buying linen

It is an economy in the long run to buy good quality linen for hotels,

Month _____ Year _____

Article	Stock in hand	New stock added	Total	Less con-demned	Total	Actual stock at stock-taking	Discrep-ancies
Sheets: single							
double							
cot							
Pillow slips							
Towels: hand							
bath							
sheet							
Table napkins							
Tablecloths: 36x36							
54x54							
54x90							
70x70							

Part of a sample page from a linen stock book

because of the great use and frequent launderings to which it is subjected. Each type of article should be chosen with regard to fibre, weave, tensile strength, washability, colour and general suitability for purpose.

Linen may be ordered direct from the manufacturers, from a large wholesale store or through a sales representative. In any case, it is advisable to get prices and see samples from more than one source, and weigh up the merits of each against the cost.

The linen for any establishment may be bought by any one of a number of senior staff, or it may be ordered from a head office when the establishment belongs to a group and there is a central buying department. When buying, the following points should be given consideration:

1 Obtain samples and test for quality and strength by:
(a) rubbing the material between the hands over dark material and noting the amount of dressing, i.e. starch, which falls on to it; if much falls it denotes a poor quality material;
(b) looking at the material under a magnifying glass to note the closeness and evenness of the weave;
(c) noting the firmness of the selvedge and the finish of the machining, especially at the corners;
(d) sending a sample of the material to the laundry to be washed a given number of times, and comparing it with a once washed sample, to get some idea of the wearing quality.
2 Buy the best quality for the purpose.
3 Buy as large a quantity at one time as possible in order to get the cheapest rates. Large orders may be given and the deliveries staggered, as the manufacturers will hold the stock until such time as it is required. This makes for cheaper buying and provided linen is stored correctly (well wrapped and perfectly dry) it will not deteriorate.
4 Buy from a reputable firm so that any complaints may be dealt with.
5 Place orders in good time so that exact requirements can be met, particularly regarding size and marking.

Firms will undertake the marking of articles at a small extra cost. Where large numbers of good quality table linen and towels are ordered, the name, initials or crest may be woven into the fabric. In other cases embroidery may be used. Embroidered names may be worked on most articles except such expendable articles as dusters and kitchen cloths.

The weaving and embroidering of the names undertaken by the manufacturers, must not be confused with machine marking done in the linen room.

Linen hire

Owing to the high cost of linen and its upkeep, the hiring of linen from firms offering a linen rental service is becoming more popular. The firms undertake to supply clean articles in good condition, and arrangements are made between the firm and the house regarding the amount of linen required, the frequency of deliveries and the price to be charged.

The advantages are:

it cuts out the heavy initial cost of buying linen;
the cost of hiring and usage is added directly to the running costs of the establishment;
linen hire charges may be no greater than the combined depreciation and laundering costs;

it cuts out the need to order new linen;

no repairing of linen on the premises is necessary;

there may be a smaller linen storage room;

fewer staff are necessary and therefore there are less wages to pay;

special sizes for staff uniforms are available;

short term loans are possible for special occasions, e.g. banqueting;

in most instances, and if stock is returned, there will be no cost to the establishment which closes for part or parts of the year.

The disadvantages are:

little choice regarding quality and style (especially of sheets);

standards not always maintained;

no rags available from the linen room;

no renovated articles, e.g. cot sheets, under pillowslips, etc.

the contract price remains the same even when numbers fall over a short period.

Amount of linen

The amount of table and bed linen required by an establishment will vary considerably, depending on the type of trade carried on. As far as bed linen is concerned, one factor to be taken into account is the frequency with which the beds are changed. A luxury hotel will re-sheet each day, other hotels will re-sheet every second or third day, while yet others only once a week and this also applies to staff quarters. In all establishments, re-sheeting is always done after a departure, and this may mean that where there are many 'one nighters', many beds will in fact be re-sheeted each day.

Another factor which will influence the amount of linen is the frequency with which the laundry collects and delivers. A good commercial laundry in a town normally takes forty-eight hours between collection and return of the articles and will pick up and deliver each day, but this does not hold good over weekends and public holidays.

Four or five times the quantity of linen required for re-sheeting, i.e. sheets, slips, towels, is the average amount necessary for most hotels. This means that for 100 beds, there may be 400 pairs of sheets which will allow 100 pairs on the beds, 100 pairs in the floor linen cupboards, 100 pairs in the linen room and 100 pairs at the laundry. This only allows for one batch of linen at the laundry at any one time, whereas in actual fact, there could be two or even three batches. Thus in some hotels five or even as much as eight times the quantity of linen in use, is more usual. Where the complete re-sheeting is once a fortnight, i.e. 1 sheet, 1 slip per week as in many hostels, the number of sheets required is 2–3 pairs.

When one considers, that for even a small establishment of perhaps

20 beds, many hundreds of articles for the bedrooms alone will be necessary, it will be realised that a great deal of money is spent on linen.

Spoilage of Linen

The following are a few reminders of the ways in which linen and its appearance may be damaged:

1   Misuse of linen by waiters and maids.
2   Insufficient care of damp and stained linen, resulting in mildew and the spread of iron mould.
3   Carelessness in stripping beds, resulting in sheets getting torn by castors.
4   Unnecessary use of bleach at the laundry.
5   Lack of adequate protection during storage, resulting in the folds becoming marked and the need for extra laundering.
6   Lack of inspection, resulting in torn articles being used and the tears becoming worse.
7   Insufficient stock and poor rotation, resulting in linen not resting between laundering and the next use.
8   Careless handling, resulting in soiling, creasing etc.

Characteristics of launderable linen

Sheets. Linen sheets are too expensive for most establishments; they crease easily and therefore require frequent laundering to keep them in good appearance; they are cold to the touch, especially in winter. They are, however, extremely hard wearing and retain a good white colour.

Cotton sheets are less expensive than linen ones, crease less easily and are warmer to the touch. They wear well and are used in the vast majority of places. They should be closely woven in a plain and well-balanced weave (i.e. little difference between the warp and the weft). The balance of threads gives the fabric its strength. The number of warp and weft ends per sq. cm. is known as the count and the higher the count, the better quality sheeting and the less potential shrinkage there is likely to be. Shrinkage may occur up to 10 washes and may be as much as 5%.

Percale sheets are made from cotton of a high quality and have a count as high as 180–200 per 6.45 cm² (per sq. inch) (whereas a good quality ordinary cotton sheet will have a count of 140–180 per 6.45 cm²) They have a smooth, soft, silky feel because combing (after carding of the fibres) removes the short fibres. Percale sheets are lighter in weight than ordinary cotton sheets and so cost less when laundered if charge is by weight. They are used in some luxury hotels (especially American). Flannelette sheets, i.e. brushed cotton, are cheaper and much warmer but have not the crisp appearance of linen or cotton.

Cotton and linen fibres are stronger wet than dry and withstand the heat and friction of laundering processes. They are not harmed by alkalis (detergents are alkaline), and will withstand, if necessary, oxidising bleaches containing chlorine when used in correct concentrations.

Sheets may be fitted to the shape of the mattress when the bottom sheet will have four corners fitted and the top sheet two. In American establishments the fitted bottom sheet is often used. They are found to be lighter in weight and cheaper than non-fitted ones of the same specification. They make a neater bed and time can be saved in smoothing and retucking especially on studio beds and when 'turning down'.

However some mending at the corners may become necessary; they are difficult to fold (they should be folded with the pockets outside to allow the air to escape); they take up more space on the shelf (1 dozen ironed stack 15 cm. high) and more work is involved in the sorting of bottom and top sheets.

Sheets made from synthetic fibres, e.g. nylon and terylene, are very hard wearing, however, they are thin and white ones tend to discolour. They do not give the same pleasing, crisp appearance of clean linen or cotton sheets; they also tend to be hot in summer and cool in winter. They are slippery and need to be fitted to the shape of the mattress, are difficult to fold and store neatly on the shelves and melt with the heat of a cigarette. Sheets from synthetic fibres are easily laundered on the premises, but cost more than cotton or linen ones when sent to a commercial laundry.

Linen and cotton union sheets are available but polyester and cotton union sheets are now much more frequently used. Originally they were 67/33 polyester/cotton but are now 50/50 and consequently not so thin. They are resin treated and so will not stand up to temperatures above 80°C. They require no ironing if folded whilst still warm from the tumble drier and their potential shrinkage is less than for a 100% cotton sheet.

Sheets should be long enough to give a good tuck in, and a good turn over at the top to protect the blankets and quilt from grease, newspaper print, the base of breakfast trays, etc. Normally for a single bed of 85 x 190 cm a single sheet should be 177 x 274 cm, for a double bed of 135 x 190 cm the sheet should be 238 x 274 cm, for a king-size bed of 182 x 200 cm the sheets need to be still larger and are frequently 274 x 297 cm.

For many years, sheets have had a wider hem at the top than at the bottom; this concentrates the wear in the same places and makes more work for the maids when making the beds and for these reasons, many establishments buy sheets with equal hems.

Pillowslips. Pillowslips will be made of the same material as the sheets. Frills and hemstitching are not recommended, and the housewife or flap type is the most usual as buttoned and taped slips need more attention regarding repairs. Even with the housewife style there is a tendency for the seam to become unstitched and establishments are now using longer slips without flaps, so that the pillow is hidden without being tucked into a flap. Slips should fit easily over the pillow and are usually 50 x 76 cm.

In order that the ticking holding the filling of the pillows should be kept clean, under pillowslips are usual. These may be of cheaper cotton or be 'remakes' from redundant sheets; they are not changed as frequently as the top pillowslips, but laundered when they become soiled.

Bath towels. Bath towels are usually of cotton in a turkish, i.e. terry weave which has a looped pile on both sides. The pile should be close for greater absorbency, and not too long or the threads will pull. The selvedge should be strong and the corners of the hems firmly stitched. The foundation cloth determines the durability of the towel. It should be strong, closely woven and when held to the light, little light should show through. A terylene foundation cloth is sometimes used for strength, but it should be realised that the use of terylene will decrease the overall absorbency of the towel. Towels with fringed ends are rarely used as hems are stronger and stand up better to the frequent launderings.

Sometimes towels are coloured, but the colours should be fast so that they may be treated as white as far as the laundry is concerned. There is a tremendous variation in the sizes of bath towels but 60 x 122 cm or 76 x 152 cm are frequently used, while larger sizes, e.g. 122 x 182 cm, are called bath sheets, and normally only used in private bathrooms.

Face and hand towels. Face and hand towels may be of linen or cotton, and in the past were always of huckaback which is a close, fancy weave but now turkish towelling hand towels are being provided in the majority of hotels. Best quality huckaback towels are very smooth and always made of linen. The usual size of a face towel is 50 x 100 cm and normally one of these and one bath towel are provided for each *guest*. For use in cloakrooms, smaller hand towels may be provided and the sizes may be 30 x 45 cm or 25 x 35 cm.

Roller towels. Roller towels may be of turkish towelling, cotton huckaback or plain woven linen. For hygienic reasons they have generally been replaced by the continuous roller towel on hire, where each person has a clean piece of towel, and are usually 40-45 cm wide.

Lavatory towels. Lavatory towels are frequently made of turkish or huckaback towelling with the word 'Toilet' woven across them, and a tape is attached for hanging. They are used for wiping the seat of the W.C. and should never be used for any other purpose. They may be 'remakes' from the linen room and the size is 35 x 45 cm approximately. Smaller disposable lavatory towels are being provided in many cloakrooms and private bathrooms.

Razor towels. Razor towels are small squares of turkish or huckaback towelling used to prevent the cutting of other towels. They may be bought or 'remakes', but in many hotels have been replaced by paper razor pads.

Bathmats. Bathmats need to be very absorbent and are often made of turkish towelling or candlewick. These are laundered frequently and so are considered more hygienic than bathmats of cork or sponge rubber. The size is 60 x 90 cm approximately. Disposable ones are available.

Table linen. Table linen may be of plain linen, but is traditionally woven in the damask weave from either linen or cotton threads. Linen cloths have a better appearance than cotton ones; they are smoother, have a natural sheen and crisper, better defined folds but they are of course much more expensive. The weave should be close with many threads to the square cm, and it may be single or double damask depending on the number of weft threads over which the warp threads pass to form the pattern. In the case of double damask there is a more well defined pattern. There are several well known designs, of which the smaller ones, e.g. the ivy and the oak leaf, giving a more all over pattern, are more economical in use. Some slipcloths are made of linen in a plain weave when they are generally coloured and coarser than the damask cloths.

Table cloths may be squares of 91 cm, 137 cm, 160 cm and 182 cm; oblongs of 131 x 182 cm, 182 x 228 cm, 182 x 320 cm and many others. It is usual to have 30 cm–45 cm overhang.

Table napkins usually match the cloths, but in some cases are in a contrasting colour, and the sizes vary from 45 cm square to 60 cm square.

Tray cloths and trolley cloths are usually of damask weave or plain linen. They are often 'remakes' from the linen room and their sizes vary.

Waiters' cloths. Waiters' cloths are usually made of white linen or cotton material, often in a basket weave. They may be bought ready made or be 'remakes' from the linen room, and are approximately 56 cm square.

Glass cloths. Glass cloths must be made from linen as cotton leaves linters on the glasses. The linen must be strong and closely woven, usually of a plain weave and the cloths often have a coloured border or central coloured stripe. They are used for table and tooth glasses. The sizes vary but they are frequently 55 x 80 cm or 65 x 90 cm.

Tea towels and kitchen rubbers. Tea towels and kitchen rubbers are similar to glass cloths but need not be of linen, and are sometimes in a twill weave.

Oven cloths. Oven cloths are often made of hessian and are of variable sizes.

4

Laundry, Dry Cleaning and the Removal of Stains

Since linen and the laundering of it is such an expensive item, it would seem sensible that anyone responsible for linen should know a little of the work done in a laundry. It is an advantage if the *housekeeper* and/or the linen keeper visits the laundry, so that misunderstandings may be prevented and good co-operation ensured.

In an establishment where linen is changed very frequently, it is more 'washed out' than 'worn out' and so the life of a sheet, for example, is often given as perhaps 200–250 washes rather than 2–3 years. But, and it is a big but, the 'life' depends on the care of the linen in use and the treatment it gets at the laundry; not forgetting that good quality material needs to be bought in the first instance.

Thus, a good laundry is of great importance to any establishment in order that:

articles are handled carefully;
tensile strength of the material is not impaired;
white material is kept white;
articles are returned clean and without any stains;
materials are not ruined by excessive use of bleach;
lists are checked carefully so that there are few 'shorts';
the work is carried out as speedily as possible;
good co-operation is maintained regarding damage and losses.

Most launderable linen is made from white cotton or linen fibres and a brief outline of the laundering is as follows:

When soiled linen arrives at the laundry it is checked and sorted into groups, then a suitable number of similar articles, e.g. sheets, are put into a

Washing machine—a large drum which revolves first in one direction and then in the other to prevent tangling of the articles. Agitation, hot water between 85°–94°C and suitable detergents (usually synthetic with a small quantity of soap added to act as a lubricant) bring about the cleansing action, after which rinsing in several waters takes place and all these processes may be automatically controlled.

Most laundries soften their water and often a 'brightener' is added to help keep whites white. Heavily soiled articles, e.g. kitchen rubbers, may need a little bleach in the washing water, but it should only be used when really necessary as it weakens the material. Table linen may need a little starch and this is added to the last rinsing water.

The clean articles are then passed into a

Hydro-extractor—which whirls the water out of the articles leaving them as a very tightly packed mass which needs shaking out in a special tumbler. There are however modern washer extractors with a dry weight capacity of about 5–400 Kg which can wash, rinse, hydro-extract and shake out all in the one machine.

The articles may now be put through a

Calender or ironing machine—This very large machine consists of several heated and well padded rollers which iron the article as it passes through. Only flat articles are calendered and a large calender will be wide enough to take a double sheet. After ironing, the articles are folded either by an automatic electric device or by hand and they are then ready for sorting, packing and despatching back to the establishment.

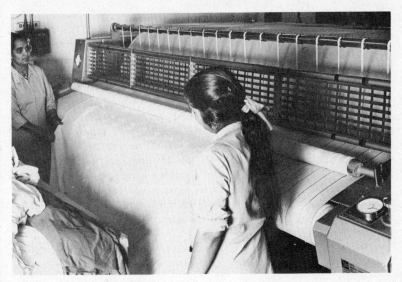

A Calender or ironing machine

In some establishments cotton and terylene blends, usually 50/50, are popular for launderable linen but these are washed at a lower temperature than all cotton articles (the resin finish is harmed above about 80°C). If not ironed, as intended they are not put into the hydro-extractor but tumble dried and folded whilst warm. This however is not possible at a commercial laundry.

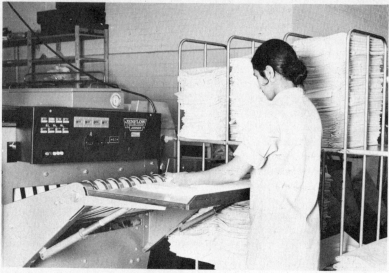

A folding machine

Shaped articles, such as shirts, nurses' uniforms, white coats, waiters' jackets, overalls, etc., cannot be ironed through a calender so they are dealt with on presses or by steam inflated 'suzies'.

Blankets are possibly the only woollen articles which an establishment sends to the laundry (they may, of course, be dry cleaned) and here the problem is to keep them fluffy. To do this, blankets should be washed in cool water (38°C) with a suitably mild detergent, a minimum amount of friction and avoiding the use of soda and bleach. They are dried on racks or put into a heated machine which tumbles them dry. Acrilan blankets may be laundered more satisfactorily than woollen ones; there is little tendency to shrink and their finish after tumble drying is excellent. Cotton cellular blankets as used in hospitals may be dealt with as for sheets.

Articles with loose colour, i.e. colours which run, such as yellow dusters, must be kept separate from other articles during the washing and drying process.

Nylon articles are very easily washed and dried and so are not often sent to the laundry, but when they are, the finish presents problems. Fitted nylon sheets when washed at home require no ironing as any rough appearance is soon lost when they are stretched on the bed. However, a laundry has to return articles with a good appearance and in order to do this, fitted nylon sheets need special care in ironing and consequently cost more than cotton or linen sheets to have laundered.

Unlined curtains and bedspreads are probably the main rayon

articles sent to the laundry and these need care in washing as rayon fibres are weak when wet and will not stand up to high temperatures.

Fresh tea and coffee stains are usually removed from white linen during the ordinary washing process, but other stains, e.g. rust and mildew, require special treatment and this is not undertaken by the laundry unless specially requested when a charge will be made. Stained articles for special treatment should therefore be sent to the laundry in a separate container.

Some large establishments have their own laundries on the premises and there are many advantages, such as no transport costs and difficulties, a quicker turnover, more freedom in laundering methods employed, fewer losses and inspection of linen can be undertaken more easily thus saving time in the linen room. However, it is only an economic proposition if the equipment is kept working to full capacity and in the past the equipment was too large and too expensive for most establishments. However it is possible these days to purchase smaller laundry equipment and the advent of 50/50 polyester/cotton bed and table linen with its non-iron finish means no calender, and so more establishments are having laundries on their premises.

Of course for a number of years some places have used domestic laundry equipment for such items as towels and articles made of synthetic fibres. There are also halls of residence, hostels and hotels where laundry facilities are provided for residents. Instead of purchasing, it is possible to hire laundry equipment but as in all cases of hiring it needs careful consideration.

Dry Cleaning

The responsibility for the sorting, despatching, receiving and storing of articles to be dry cleaned may be that of the linen keeper or an assistant housekeeper.

In addition to the dry cleaning of blankets, curtains, quilts, etc., some staff have a dry cleaning allowance for their 'working dress'. In an hotel, guests' dry cleaning is despatched by the valet, hall porter or the linen keeper. Articles for dry cleaning may be sent to a firm of dry cleaners or to a laundry with a dry cleaning department.

On arrival at the cleaners, each article is marked with an identifying tape, checked for special stains and items in the pockets, and brushed free of loose dust. Certain types of stains such as blood, paint, lipstick, etc., are removed more easily if some attention is given to them before cleaning, so these stain areas are 'pre-spotted'.

Although in certain instances different coloured articles may be cleaned successfully together, it is normal to divide the work into a number of classifications such as whites, mediums, darks, etc., so that heavily soiled articles are not cleaned with lighter soiled ones and dark coloured lint does not then transfer to light coloured articles or vice versa.

The prepared articles are then 'washed' in a dry cleaning solvent, such as perchlorethylene, in an enclosed machine in which the washing, extraction and drying is all carried out in the same cage. The solvent, because of its cost, is not wasted, but distilled and/or filtered for re-use.

Dry cleaning solvents do not affect textile fibres in the same way as water, and so when cleaning some materials the risk of shrinkage or severe creasing, distortion, colour movement, etc., may be greatly reduced. (N.B. Shrinkage may occur partly because of the agitation and partly because a small amount of water may be present.) Because water borne soil and stains can only effectively be removed by the use of water, a controlled amount of water and detergent is introduced into the solvent during some dry cleaning processes (known as 'charged system'). After the articles have been cleaned in a series of solvent washes, they are spun dried to extract the bulk of the solvent and then dried with warm air. The cleaned articles are hung up and checked for stains; any remaining are dealt with before pressing.

After pressing, the articles are returned in hampers, boxes or on coat hangers and in the case of guests' dry cleaning, the cost is entered on to the individual account.

Stain Removal

Many fresh stains, e.g. tea, coffee, grease, etc., will be removed from cotton and linen articles during the normal washing process. Protein stains, e.g. egg, blood, glue, perspiration, etc., are more easily removed by pre-soaking in lukewarm water with a detergent containing enzymes which digest the protein. (N.B. Enzymes are inactive in hot water.)

Stains, if old or heavy, require special treatment with stain removal agents. The use of these stain removal agents requires care as they can cause weakening of the fibres, bleeding of dyes, damage to special fabric finishes, and some are inflammable while others are poisonous. The main stain removal agents are:

1   *Organic solvents*, e.g. (*a*) benzine, white spirit (turpentine substitute), amyl acetate, acetone, methylated spirit; (*b*) carbon tetrachloride, perchlorethylene.

These dissolve grease and require care in use because some (the (*a*) group) are inflammable and should never be used near a naked flame, and others (the (*b*) group), while they are non-inflammable, are harmful when inhaled and should be used only in a well ventilated area.

The majority of these solvents will not harm fibres or dyes but there are exceptions. For example, acetone dissolves rayon acetate, and amyl acetate, though not so active, is safer; others affect rubber (rubber backed carpets), etc.

Chewing gum (after scraping), grease, oil paint, lipstick, ball-point ink, etc., will sometimes yield to a solvent.

2 *Acids*, e.g. oxalic acid, potassium acid oxalate (salts of lemon), and various rust removers sold under trade names. [All these are poisonous.]

Fibres vary in their susceptibility to damage by acids; however, dilute acids can be used on most white fabrics. Some dyes may be affected by acids which therefore should only be used on fast colours. Washing, using a detergent, or thorough rinsing in a weak alkaline solution is essential to neutralise the acid and prevent damage to the fabric after treatment, as any remaining acid becomes more concentrated during the drying process. Always remember that alkalis affect animal fibres.

Acids will dissolve a wide variety of metals and are therefore of use in removing metal stains, the commonest of which are iron mould or rust, and the iron stain left after washing a blood-stained article. Any of the acids mentioned above are suitable for the removal of rust from any white fabric, but it is better to repeat the treatment several times rather than use a concentrated solution.

3 *Alkalis*, e.g. soda, borax, ammonia.

Old and heavy vegetable stains e.g. tea, coffee, wine etc. are removed by alkalis from white linen and cotton fabrics. Dyes and animal fibres may be adversely affected by alkalis.

4 *Bleaches*. The process of changing a coloured substance into a colourless one is known as bleaching, i.e. bleaches whiten. Bleaches also weaken fibres so extreme care is needed in their use. They whiten by either oxidising or reducing the coloured substance.

(*a*) Oxidising bleaches liberate oxygen from themselves or other substances and the most frequently used oxidising bleaches are sodium hypochlorite, hydrogen peroxide and sodium perborate.

Sodium hypochlorite (normal household bleach) damages animal fibres and so should not be used on woollen or silk articles. It is used mainly for the removal of obstinate stains on cotton and linen fabrics but it 'fixes' iron stains. All fabrics should be thoroughly rinsed after being treated with hypochlorites or rotting of the fabrics will occur. An added hazard with 50/50 polyester/cotton fabrics is that the resin tends to retain the chlorine. In commercial use, an anti-chlor, e.g. sodium thiosulphate ('hypo') is added to the final rinse to remove all traces of the free chlorine.

Hydrogen peroxide is slower acting than the hypochlorite bleaches and can be used on most white fabrics. The peroxide decomposes more readily if the solution is rendered just alkaline with ammonia.

Sodium perborate is the bleach present in powdered soap and soapless detergents. It is safe to use on most fabrics and is quick acting at high temperatures.

(*b*) Reducing bleaches remove oxygen or add hydrogen to the coloured substance and sodium hydrosulphite is the most frequently used. It can be used on most white fabrics and is used for the removal of iron stains and the stripping of dyes. It is in general, milder in its action than the oxidising bleaches. White articles bleached by reduction e.g. woollen blankets, straw mats, are liable to take up oxygen in sunlight and become yellowed.

5   *Enzymes*, e.g. powdered pepsin, may be used for the removal of protein stains on all fabrics.

If the origin of a stain is known then the specific stain removal agent can be used straight away, but if unknown, it may be necessary to try several agents before the right one is found. In general, safer treatments are tried first. For this reason, it is better to repeat a process twice with a weak solution than to use a strong solution at the beginning, and in any case, it is essential that the agents are completely removed from the fabric by neutralisation, washing or thorough rinsing.

Stains on coloured materials are very difficult to remove as many of the stain removal agents affect dyes. In the case of carpets and upholstery, stains are particularly difficult to remove because they have to be dealt with *in situ*, and the colour, the backing and padding may present problems. Grease absorbers in the form of aerosol sprays may prove useful.

It must be strongly emphasised that stain removal, owing to the variety of fibres used in modern materials and the unknown qualities of some stains, is a highly skilled job and should not be undertaken lightly.

Fabrics may be treated so as to be made 'stain repellent' and this may be achieved by the use of fluorochemicals e.g. Scotchgard which will give both water and oil repellency. The stains tend to stand on the surface and can be blotted away (not wiped). These finishes are expensive but there is no change in colour or texture of the fabric and they withstand dry cleaning and at least five washes.

Much more usually the fabrics are made water repellent only, by the use of silicones when water borne stains will not wet the surface and so can be blotted away. The fabric will still absorb oil-borne stains but even they are more easily removed with solvent cleansers which do not remove the silicone finish.

Polyurethane is sometimes used as a very thin flexible coating on some fabrics intended to be waterproof.

Specific stain removal agents—for the more usual stains on white and fast-coloured fabrics:

Ball-point ink: Methylated spirit or carbon tetrachloride.
Blood (stain left after washing): Treat as for *iron mould*.
Dyes: Bleach (not chlorine bleaches on animal fibres).
Grass: Methylated spirit.
Ink: If not removed by washing treat as for *iron mould*.
Ink (red): Often not removable, except when very fresh, but some may
    respond to washing or sodium hydrosulphite.

Iron mould: Rust remover, oxalic acid, potassium acid oxalate (salts of lemon), or sodium hydrosulphite.

Lacquer and nail varnish: Amyl acetate, acetone (not on rayon acetate) or a cellulose thinner.

Lipstick: Carbon tetrachloride and/or sodium hydrosulphite.

Mildew: Hot weak potassium permanganate solution followed by a weak acid or hydrogen peroxide.

Paint (oil): If fresh, white spirit, or a proprietary paint remover followed by a solvent.

Paint (cellulose): Amyl acetate, acetone (not on rayon acetate) or a commercial cellulose thinner.

Paint (emulsion): Wash immediately, as once dried it is almost irremovable.

Perspiration: Treat as for mildew or protein stains.

Protein stains, e.g. egg, meat, perspiration: Protein digesting enzyme, e.g. pepsin.

Tar: Carbon tetrachloride or white spirit, scraping first.

Vegetable stains, e.g. tea, coffee, etc.: Alkali or bleach (not chlorine bleaches on animal fibres).

The removal of stains from a variety of surfaces:

Carpets and upholstery (care must be taken not to wet the backing or padding)

Candle grease: Scrape, use hot iron and absorbent paper. Followed if necessary with a grease solvent.

Ink: Mop up as quickly as possible to prevent spreading. Wash with warm water and synthetic detergent or use a weak acid, and rinse.

Mud: Leave to dry, then brush off

Shoe polish: Scrape off if possible and then apply a grease solvent.

Urine: Sponge with salt water, followed by a weak solution of ammonia and rinse well.

Polished wood

Ink: Mop up as quickly as possible. Rub with fine dry steel wool or glass paper, or dab with a hot solution of weak acid and rinse. In both cases colour and polish will be removed, so rub with linseed oil or shoe polish to darken and later apply polish, and buff well.

Spills, slight heat and burn marks: Rub with a rag moistened with a drop or two of liquid metal polish or methylated spirit and then repolish, or rub with a very fine abrasive, e.g. cigarette ash or very fine steel wool and repolish.

Scratch marks: Cover with iodine, potassium permanganate solution or shoe polish according to the colour of the wood.

Wood with oil finish

Small burns and heat marks: Rub with emery cloth or fine sandpaper, followed by boiled linseed oil.

Marble, terrazzo

Ink: Apply a poultice of sodium perborate, precipitated whiting and
water. Leave to dry.

Rust: Apply a poultice of sodium citrate crystals, glycerine, precipitated
whiting and water. Leave to dry.

Points to remember in stain removal:

1 Treat stains as soon as possible.
2 Consider the fibres of which the fabric is made.
3 If a coloured article, check effect of remover on an unimportant
part if possible.
4 Use the weakest methods first.
5 Use a weak solution several times, rather than one strong one.
6 After using a chemical, neutralise or rinse well.

5

Fabrics

Fabrics are used in a great variety of ways throughout an establishment, and may be chosen for their decorative value, for their comfort, warmth or coolness, their protective qualities, their durability and even for hygienic reasons.

As the purpose for which fabrics are required varies, so does the wear and tear put on them; they may be subjected to much soiling, and the consequent frequent launderings, to abrasion, or the possibility of snagging, creasing or fading. It is therefore essential, if the maximum use is to be obtained from these fabrics, that they are chosen with a view to the purpose for which they are required. The suitability for a particular purpose, will depend on the raw materials from which the fabrics are made and on the method of manufacture.

Basically, fabrics are made from fibres which may be natural—cotton, linen, wool and silk being the most frequently used natural fibres, or man-made, for example, rayon, nylon, terylene and acrilan. These fibres are twisted (spun) into long threads (yarn), from which the majority of fabrics are manufactured but there are, however, fabrics produced directly from fibres. The physical and chemical properties of the fibres will have great bearing on the characteristics of the fabrics containing them. Thus, for example, the softness, strength, elasticity, lustre and the resistance to wear of the fabric as well as any treatments such as dyeing, crease and shrinkage resistance, which may be given to the yarn or the fabric, will depend on the properties of the basic fibre or fibres and as new fibres and treatments become available so the problems of fading, creasing, wear and general maintenance become less. As the same or different fibres may be spun together, and the threads so produced may be fine, thick, fancy, smooth or hairy, these too, will influence the characteristics of the final fabric.

In the majority of cases, the fabric is produced by the threads being woven together; however some may be knitted and there are newer fabrics produced directly from fibres by fibre bonding and similar techniques. These 'non-woven' fabrics are produced more cheaply than by weaving and have different characteristics; one particular use is for disposable and short life articles. With woven fabrics, the weave may be open or close, plain or figured and this also will affect the appearance and characteristics of the finished fabric.

Natural Fibres

Of the most frequently used natural fibres, cotton and linen are of vegetable origin, while silk and wool are of animal origin.

Vegetable fibres

These are made of cellulose; they are strong, absorbent and good conductors of heat. They launder well, are stronger wet than dry and withstand a fairly high temperature. They are generally not harmed by alkalis but lose strength in contact with acids, and have little resilience. They are mothproof but are attacked by mildew if left in a damp condition.

Cotton is the most frequently used natural fibre, and is obtained from the seed of the cotton plant. The length of the fibre varies from 1.5 cm–5 cm, and the longest fibres come from the West Indian and Egyptian cotton plants, and the shortest from American and Indian plants. West Indian cotton, when spun and woven, produces a very fine fabric, Sea Island cotton, which is frequently used for dress materials. Egyptian cotton is used for tight, fine yarns suitable for the highest grade furnishing fabrics and for bed linen, while American and Indian cottons are used for furnishing fabrics of ordinary quality. The very short cotton fibres are called cotton linters and these are not spun into yarn, but used in cotton felt for bedding and upholstery, or in the production of rayon.

Cotton fibres are flat and ribbonlike, and have a natural twist which aids the spinning and makes a strong thread (i.e. it has good tensile strength).

Cotton fibres are good conductors of heat, but they have a slight hairiness and the air held between the 'hair' is a bad conductor, so cotton materials have a slight feeling of warmth, and this may be increased when the material is brushed or teased since more air is then held. The hairiness of the fibre accounts for cotton materials being unsuitable for polishing glass, as linters or 'bits' are left on the surface, and for materials soiling more easily than ones made from smoother fibres, e.g. linen.

Cotton has little resilience so creases occur in the fabrics made from it, and cotton yarn used for the pile of carpets soon has a flattened appearance.

Mercerised cotton is produced by treating the yarn or fabric with caustic soda, under conditions where the fibres are stretched. Mercerisation results in smoother, more rodlike fibres which have a gloss or sheen, and it gives cotton a greater affinity for dyes and improves its strength.

Linen is obtained from the stem of the flax plant, and the fibres vary between ½–1 m in length. The length of the fibre enables a fine, strong yarn to be spun.

The fibres are smooth, straight and almost solid, and these factors account for the chief differences between cotton and linen fabrics. The smoothness of the fibres gives good dirt and abrasion resistance, so linen fabrics are popular for loose covers; it also accounts for the lack of linters, and consequent suitability of linen for glass cloths, and for the fabric being cool to the touch. The smoothness and the straightness of the fibres give linen its lustre, which can be increased by mercerisation, when its strength and dye affinity are also increased. The solidity of the fibres makes linen much heavier than cotton, and the weight of a pile of linen table cloths or sheets on a shelf can be considerable.

Linen has little resilience and creases badly, the creases being much more sharply defined than in cotton fabrics—linen sheets become crumpled very much sooner than cotton ones.

Thread spun from the shorter linen fibres is known as tow yarn, and this yarn produces a soft, less 'rigid' and more absorbent material than that spun from the longer fibres, line yarn; tow yarn is therefore more suitable for towels, glass cloths, and fabrics which need to drape well. Line yarn produces a strong material with more resistance to dirt and abrasion, and is used for table linen, sheets and upholstery.

Jute, ramie, hemp and sisal are also natural fibres of vegetable origin, the first three coming from the stems of plants and the last from the leaves of a plant, but they are not used in fabrics to the same extent as cotton and linen.

Jute, hemp and sisal are used for twines and sacks; jute is also used for hessian, and the backing of carpets and linoleum; sisal is used for the manufacture of mats when it is now often used in conjunction with plastic threads. Although the main use of hemp is for twines, canvas and sacks, it can be made into lustrous fabrics. Ramie is very strong and has a fine natural lustre, and was used in high grade furnishing fabrics, especially pile fabrics, but owing to difficulties, mainly in supply, it is not used so much now.

Kapok is obtained from the seed of the kapok tree. The fibre is smooth, light and lustrous. It is used for the filling of pillows and cushions, especially by people with an allergy to feathers, but it has been replaced in many instances by rubber or plastic foam or synthetic fibres e.g. terylene.

Animal fibres

These are made of protein, and there is a great variation in the physical form and structure of the different fibres. They are, however, soft, absorbent and poor conductors of heat. They disintegrate in sunlight and are damaged by heat. They are fairly resistant to acids but are harmed by alkalis and chlorine bleaches. They have elasticity and resilience.

Wool normally means the fibre from the fleece of the sheep, but fibres from other animals, e.g. horse, camel, llama, and goats are also used. Most wool is the yearly growth from the living animal, that is, fleece or virgin wool, but 'skin' or 'pulled' wool may be obtained from the bodies of dead sheep, and remanufactured wools may be obtained from used wool. Of the remanufactured wools, 'shoddy' is perhaps the best for re-use, and it is obtained when knitted woollens, flannels and worsted rags are run through garnetting machines which pull out the wool fibres, and these may then be respun and made up into cheaper woollen articles.

Wool fibres vary in length from about 4–40 cm and they also vary in diameter, some being very much finer than others. They have a natural crimp or wave, and this gives wool its elasticity and resilience, enabling it to resist crushing, and making it particularly suitable for carpets and upholstery. The fibres are not smooth but have overlapping scales which enable air to be held between the fibres, and woollen material to feel warm.

These scales interlock with friction, as for example in careless laundering, and bring about felting and shrinkage when the material will be less warm. In cut pile carpets, this felting is an advantage as the loose fibres, produced as a result of the cutting of the pile yarn, become bedded down in the carpet.

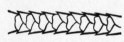

A woollen fibre

Wool fibres are used to give woollen or worsted yarns. In woollen yarns, the fibres lie in all directions and result in a hairy fabric, but for worsted yarns the fibres are combed parallel and the fabric produced from these smoother, more tightly twisted threads, is less rough and hairy, and is more expensive.

Wool cannot be dyed to the same standards of uniformity or fastness as vegetable and man-made fibres, and unlike these it is attacked by moth. Wool can be mothproofed, but care must be taken to see that the proofing withstands any cleaning process.

Silk is obtained from the cocoon spun by the cultivated silkworm, in the form of long filaments which may be on an average 274–456 metres long. The cocoon may consist of up to 3 Km of filament, but this cannot be unwound continuously.

The filaments are smooth and tubelike, with no irregularities and the beautiful lustre of silk fabrics is due to these properties. Silk is stronger than cotton (i.e. it has greater tensile strength); it is elastic and resilient and so it does not crush easily. It is, however, weakened when wet, and it disintegrates in sunlight.

Spun silk is manufactured from the shorter filaments obtained during the 'reeling' or unwinding of the cocoons, or from pierced cocoons, and it is less smooth and lustrous than thrown silk made from the finest filaments.

Silkworms of the wild silk moth, such as the Tussah moth, feed at will in the open, on leaves of various trees, and produce wild silk. The filaments are frequently irregular, producing slubs or variations in thickness when the silk is woven and the natural gum is not completely removed as is the case in silk from the cultivated silkworm.

All silk materials have elegance but due to their expense, their use is normally confined to luxury establishments.

Asbestos

In addition to natural fibres of vegetable and animal origin there is a mineral one, asbestos. It occurs naturally in many parts of the world; it is quite incombustible and is used for fireproof materials, and as a filler in certain types of floorings.

Man-made Fibres

The number of man-made fibres has increased tremendously in recent years, and there can be no doubt that still more and improved fibres will be discovered as research continues. All man-made fibres are manufactured in basically the same way. The raw materials are treated chemically to form a viscous liquid, after which long continuous filaments are produced, in varying thicknesses depending on the size of the spinning jet used. The long filaments may be cut up into fibres of required lengths, and yarns from these cut-up or staple fibres produce a less shiny fabric, with a softer and warmer handle than the continuous filament yarns. Some staple fibres may be 'bulked' to give an even warmer handle, and improved absorbency. Man-made fibres are mothproof and the majority are mildew proof and have a low moisture absorbency.

Man-made fibres may be *regenerated*, for example, rayon, when the fibres are retrieved from natural substances, the most usual being cellulose, or *synthetic*, for example, nylon, when the fibres are produced by chemical synthesis (i.e. they are built up from basic chemicals).

Regenerated fibres

Rayon. The term 'rayon' often covers viscose, acetate and cuprammonium fibres, but while viscose and cuprammonium rayons have many properties in common, they differ considerably from rayon acetate. It would, therefore, seem wiser to restrict the term rayon to viscose rayon, as is more usual in America. Cuprammonium rayon has not the importance of viscose and acetate rayons in the field of furnishing fabrics, and will not be considered here.

Viscose rayon filaments consist of pure regenerated cellulose obtained from wood pulp or cotton linters. As cotton, the filaments have little resilience, and so viscose rayon flattens when used in carpets, and creases badly. It absorbs water better than cotton, has a lowered wet strength, is more receptive to dyes and is harmed more easily by bleaches and other chemicals. It decomposes without melting at 185°–222°C. As the filaments are smooth, yarn and fabrics made from them have a lustre and are inclined to lose their shape especially when wet.

The basic properties of viscose rayon can be modified during manufacture and a number of modified rayon fibres are available.

Evlan, a modified viscose rayon fibre, because of its improved durability and resilience was developed especially for carpets and is used in blends for tufted and woven carpets as well as in 100 per cent. form. It is also used extensively in upholstery fabrics. Evlan M is an improved version and Evlan FR is flame resistant.

Vincel of all the rayons resembles cotton most closely, and provides a high resistance to shrinkage. It is frequently used in blends with other man-made and natural fibres giving the fabrics an appearance of high quality cotton.

Sarille is the modified rayon with a high degree of crimp and so produces fabrics with a wool-like handle. It has crease shedding properties and is used for blankets and candlewick bedspreads when it has the advantage of being lint free.

Durafil, because of its improved durability and resistance to abrasion, can be used in blends for uniform and upholstery fabrics.

Rayon acetate is also obtained from wood pulp or cotton linters, but as it is a cellulose derivative and not cellulose, it has different properties from viscose rayon. Rayon acetate is not as absorbent as viscose rayon; it becomes softened at 180°C and melts at 230°C; it is soluble in various organic solvents, e.g. acetone, and is harmed by acids and alkalis.

Rayon triacetate has a low moisture absorbency and therefore tends to accumulate an electrostatic charge. It has the same wet and dry strength as rayon acetate but it is more crease shedding and has a higher melting point, about 260°C, and is not harmed as easily by alkalis. It is harmed by trichlorethylene and so must not be dry cleaned in this solvent; perchlorethylene can, however, be used. Triacetate is used for the pile and backing of candlewick fabrics and may be 'bulked' and used as the filling for quilts.

Neither viscose nor acetate rayon is suitable for furnishing fabrics which require constant laundering. Rayon acetate has the softer handle, and the fabric drapes well and is more silklike, but it should only be used where it is not subjected to great strain, for example, lightweight curtains and bedspreads. Rayon is frequently blended with other fibres of greater strength, and the fabric can then be used for upholstery, loose covers and heavy curtains.

Fibrolane is a regenerated protein fibre from casein, and it has wool-like properties. It is warm, light and soft, absorbent, resilient and crease resistant.

Fibrolane is mixed with other fibres normally because of its low strength especially when wet, and it is used to some extent in the manufacture of carpets.

Other regenerated protein fibres are obtained from proteins extracted from corn, ground nuts and soya beans, but these fibres have relatively little importance, compared with the other man-made fibres.

Synthetic fibres

Synthetic fibres may be grouped according to their chemical composition, for example:

Polyamide fibres, e.g. nylon
polyester fibres, e.g. terylene
acrylic fibres, e.g. acrilan
polyvinyl fibres, e.g. saran

polyolefin fibres $\begin{cases} \text{polyethylene, e.g. courlene} \\ \text{polypropylene, e.g. ulstron} \end{cases}$

Their individual names, however, prove confusing as different manufacturers give their own trade names to fibres of similar properties; thus Perlon is the German brand of nylon, and Dacron the American terylene.

Most synthetic fibres are produced as continuous filaments which may be cut into staple form; these may, in some cases, be 'bulked' to give a softer and warmer handle. Bulked fibres tend to 'pill' (i.e. the nap forms tiny balls) especially in laundering, and once the nap has gone the article is not as warm. Synthetic fibres are thermoplastic and poor conductors of heat; they have strength, elasticity, low moisture absorbency and resistance to abrasion, moth and mildew. They are electrostatic although epitropic fibres with antistatic and electrically conductive properties have now been produced. For sheer strength nylon is the best, but for ease of cleaning and resilience the acrylics are better.

Nylon is a polyamide fibre and is produced in various forms with melting points varying from 185°C to 250°C e.g. the heat from cigarette ends. There is a modified nylon produced in America which withstands high temperatures and will ignite with difficulty only at 538°C. It is however too expensive for general use.

Nylon is not normally harmed by dilute chemicals and does not crease easily, but when creases appear, they are difficult to remove. Nylon is electrostatic and so attracts dirt, and should be washed frequently; it is, however, easy to wash and dry, because of its low moisture absorbency. Its great strength, elasticity and abrasion resistance make it very suitable for upholstery fabrics and carpets.

Nylon can be brushed or 'bulked' when more air will be held between the fibres, and the fabrics will feel warmer, e.g. brushed nylon sheets.

Terylene is a polyester fibre. It melts at 243°C and has a very low moisture absorbency which makes dyeing difficult and terylene more electrostatic than nylon or the acrylics. It has a very good resistance to abrasion which even so, is inferior to nylon. Creases hold more readily than in nylon, and as terylene has a greater resistance to sunlight it is frequently used for net curtains.

Terylene is more often 'bulked' than nylon, and it is then used for the fillings of pillows and quilts. It is used in blends of 33% cotton and more recently 50% cotton for bed and table linen when little or no ironing is necessary.

Acrilan is an acrylic fibre used in staple form. It is the most wool-like of the synthetic fibres having a fluffy, soft warm handle, good resilience and crease recovery. It absorbs little moisture, melts at 246°C and has good resistance to chemicals and sunlight. It is less resistant to abrasion than nylon and terylene but it is better than wool.

It is used for blankets, upholstery fabrics and in the manufacture of carpets.

Orlon is an acrylic fibre and has properties similar to Acrilan, except that it has excellent resistance to sunlight, and is therefore very suitable for curtain fabrics.

Courtelle is also an acrylic fibre with similar properties to Acrilan; however, it does not melt but sticks to a hot iron about 154°C. It readily takes a permanent twist and is therefore particularly suitable for 'kinky' or twisted pile carpets. It is also used for blankets.

Dralon is an acrylic fibre with properties similar to Acrilan and is being used for curtain and upholstery fabrics and in the manufacture of carpets.

Teklan is a modified acrylic. It is a flameproof fibre and is used for carpets, curtains and upholstery fabrics.

Saran is a polyvinyl fibre. It is almost completely non-absorbent and therefore difficult to dye. Saran does not burn but loses strength in boiling water and softens at $121\,^\circ$C. It is used for certain types of upholstery fabrics and deck-chair coverings.

Courlene is a polyethylene fibre. It is non-absorbent, and the fibres soften about $95\,^\circ$C (i.e. below the temperature of boiling water) and melt about $120\,^\circ$C. It is used for certain types of deck-chair, awning and upholstery fabrics as well as plastic floor mattings.

Polypropylene fibres are lightest in weight of synthetic fibres, have greatest abrasion resistance and are used in some of the adhesively bonded felted carpets.

Glass fibre is produced in the form of fine filaments from molten glass. It is non-absorbent, highly resistant to chemicals and strong sunlight and it is fireproof (melting point $815\,^\circ$C).

Glass fibre has a poor resistance to abrasion; the fibres are brittle but when fine they can be woven into fabrics for light weight curtains, and for shower curtains. It is in some instances reinforced with polyester resins, and produced as a laminated sheet material which has great strength and durability, and is used for baths, lavatory basins and sinks (see Chapter 15).

The identification of textile fibres has become very complicated with the advent of so many man-made fibres (there are already over 200 registered fibres) and the increasing use of fibre mixtures, and the special treatments given to some fibres, have added to the difficulties.

It is possible, however, to examine:

1 Appearance, feel and length;
2 Appearance under the microscope;
3 Behaviour to heat and flame;
4 Behaviour and solubility in certain acids, alkalis and organic solvents;
5 Reaction to colour staining solutions, such as Shirlastain.

Fabrics

The threads spun from the fibres may be knitted or woven into a fabric or material.

During knitting, one thread is normally used to form a series or row of loops, which in turn, is held by another row and in this way stocking stitch and other stitches are formed.

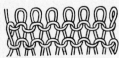

In weaving, there must be two sets of threads. The loom is set up or 'strung', with long vertical threads called the warp, and crossing or interlacing these threads, is the weft. This weft thread is carried by a shuttle, and turns at the side of the series of warp threads to form a firm edge, the selvedge.

A mixture indicates that a fabric is manufactured from two or more different yarns, e.g. a woven fabric with a nylon warp and a rayon or cotton weft.

A blend means that the fabric is made from yarns spun from two or more types of fibres.

To show the selvedge

By mixing and blending, a far greater variety of textures and colour effects can be introduced into fabrics, and fabrics may be given improved properties, e.g. greater strength, better drape or washability, etc.

Household fabrics are normally woven, that is they are textiles. Many widths of materials may be produced. The appearance, quality and behaviour in use of any fabric are dependent on the nature of the weave, as well as on the type of fibre used in the threads. Hence, some fabrics are more suitable for some purposes than others.

In the manufacture of textiles there are several standard weaves, e.g. plain, twill, satin, huckaback, damask, pile, etc.

Plain weave. In a plain weave, the weft goes over and under alternate warp threads, as in darning.

Fabrics made in a plain weave are normally smooth, and their firmness will depend on the number of warp and weft threads per cm, that is, on the closeness of the weave. A close weave gives a strong cloth, but one which tears easily. The weight and appearance of plain weave fabrics vary enormously according to the thickness, character and

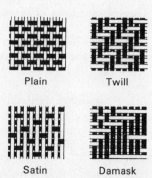

Plain Twill

Satin Damask

closeness of the threads, none of which need be the same for warp and weft.

Chintz, cretonne, scrim and sheeting are fabrics made in a plain weave. Repp and taffeta are also plain weave fabrics where the ribbed effect has been produced by using warp and weft of differing thicknesses.

Twill weave. In a twill weave, the weft threads cross the warp at different intervals in the different rows, so that a series of diagonal lines is produced on the surface of the fabrics.

Herringbone patterns are produced by reversing the direction of the twill, at regular intervals across the width of the cloth. In a twill weave the threads are normally close together, and the finished fabric is firm and hard wearing.

Twill sheeting, drill and gaberdine are fabrics made in a twill weave.

Satin weave. In a satin weave, there are fewer intersections of the warp and weft threads, and the intersections are uniformly distributed. The warp 'floats' over, for example, four weft threads and forms the surface of the fabric, i.e. the fabric is warp faced.

The fabric is smooth, usually of dense construction and with an attractive sheen. Owing to the 'floating' threads, it may present little resistance to abrasion and become pulled or snagged.

There are many types of furnishing satins, that is, furnishing fabrics made in a satin weave, e.g. cotton satin, rayon satin, etc.

A sateen weave is similar to a satin weave but it is the weft threads which 'float' and the fabric is therefore weft faced.

Figured weaves. Figured weaves are those which introduce a pattern into the fabric. The pattern may be introduced by combining two of the previously mentioned weaves, as in damask, or it may be introduced by the use of coloured threads additional to the foundation cloth, as in brocade or tapestry. Huckaback and brocatelle are other fabrics woven in a figured weave.

In all these cases, the weaves are produced on a Jacquard loom, where each warp thread is controlled individually; the thread as it is required is lifted by a harness, controlled by a series of punched cards corresponding to the pattern to be woven.

Fabrics made in figured weaves vary considerably in weight and appearance.

Pile weave. In a pile weave, there are tufts or loops of yarn which stand up from the body of the cloth. The tufts or loops are extra warp or weft threads woven at right angles through the foundation cloth. These extra threads form the pile or surface thickness, and they may be cut or uncut. Patterns can be produced by combining cut and uncut piles.

A thick, hard wearing fabric results which has a tendency to 'sprout', snag and collect dust.

Velvet is a cut, warp pile fabric; turkish (terry) towelling is an uncut pile fabric and the pile is on both sides of the material; moquette may be either a cut or uncut pile fabric.

Pile fabrics may also be made by *tufting*, e.g. candlewick.

Characteristics and Uses of the More Usual Fabrics

In some cases, certain fibres were originally associated with particular fabrics, but this is no longer the case, and many fabrics are obtainable in the different natural and man-made fibres. For example, satin was originally always made from silk but now cotton, rayon and nylon satins are available.

Alpaca. A slightly shiny, 'woollen' cloth having an alpaca or mohair weft and a cotton warp. It is frequently used for valets' waistcoats.

Armure. A fabric with a small, often self-coloured, design formed where warp and weft threads do not interlace (as in satin weave). The design appears as floating warp threads on the surface of the cloth, and it must inevitably be small or the fabric will be loose and become pulled out of shape easily. It is used for curtains and upholstery.

Baize. An all wool fabric, piece dyed, in which the surface has been raised and close cropped. It is generally green in colour and used for aprons, storing silver and covering meeting and board room tables. A very fine quality is used for billiard tables.

Barathea. A hard wearing woollen fabric, often of twill weave, used for suits and tailored uniforms.

Brocade. A patterned fabric which has extra weft threads to the normal warp and weft, introduced during the weaving. These appear on the surface of the cloth where necessary to give colour and form the pattern. Originally brocade was an all silk fabric and the coloured threads were only introduced in short lengths, as required by the design. Today the fabric is often made from cotton and man-made fibres, and coloured threads are caught in, and carried across the back from selvedge to selvedge, when not required on the surface. Brocade is used for upholstery, curtains and bedspreads.

Brocatelle. A heavy fabric in which the self-coloured pattern and the background are formed by warp satin and plain weaves respectively;

there are additional weft threads which pad the pattern, and the fabric therefore has an embossed effect. It is used for upholstery and cushion covers.

Bump. A thick fabric made of flannelette and used as an interlining for heavy curtains.

Candlewick. A fabric in which thick tufted yarns are inserted into a plain weave foundation cloth. Originally, the wick for candles, 'candlewick' was used as the tufted yarn but now thick threads of cotton or viscose rayon, and more recently sarille, triacetate, nylon or courtelle which are lint free, are used. It is used for bedspreads, and where made of cotton, rayon, sarille or triacetate for bathmats.

Calico. Any cotton material, thicker than muslin, in a plain weave. It is often left unbleached and used as dust covers for linen.

Cellular fabric. A fabric woven in such a way that there is a great deal of air held between the threads, for example cellular blankets.

Chintz. A printed cotton fabric of plain weave, with a glazed finish. Originally the pattern was very small, but it is not necessarily so today. It is used for curtains and loose covers.

Coated Cloths. Woven, knitted or bonded fibre cloths may be coated with PVC or polyurethane. The woven base gives strength and dimensional stability. A knitted base fabric is especially suitable for upholstery as it can be stretched over the curved surfaces better. These coated fabrics are usually impermeable to air and water vapour but porous coatings have been developed which give upholstery a more comfortable feel.

Corduroy. A weft pile fabric as velveteen but the cut pile forms lines or cords which run in the warp direction.

Crash. A thick, plain woven linen fabric (though now often cotton or jute) made from coarse uneven weft yarns which produce an uneven surface.

Cretonne. A printed cotton or rayon fabric of plain (sometimes twill) weave, often with horizontal ribbing. It is a coarser fabric than chintz with rather a dull finish, and originally it had a bold pattern. The name is frequently applied to linen fabrics but these should more strictly be called 'printed linens'. It is hard wearing and used for curtains and loose covers.

Damask. A figured fabric which, when used for table linen, has the figure or design in weft and the background in warp satin weaves. Both single and double damasks are used for table linen. In single damask, the satin weave is produced by one warp thread going over four and under one weft thread whereas in double damask the warp thread goes over seven or more, and under one weft, and the warp threads are frequently finer than the weft giving a closer, stronger fabric although this is not necessarily so. The essential difference is that the double damask weave gives a clearer design.

Furnishing damasks are frequently woven in warp satin and plain weaves (instead of warp and weft faced satins as in table linen), and in some instances, the design is further emphasised by the use of different fibres for the warp and weft threads. Cotton, linen, silk, rayon, nylon, terylene or any combination of these may be used; there is consequently a great variety in the weight of the fabric. Damask is probably one of the most useful furnishing fabrics, and is used for upholstery, curtains and loose covers.

Denim. A heavy cotton fabric, in which the warp is dyed and the weft undyed, so giving a speckled effect, often bluey-grey. It is very hard wearing and used for overalls.

Drill. A heavy, cotton fabric similar to denim, but the warp and weft are either both left white, or both dyed when the fabric is often buff coloured. It is very hard wearing and used for overalls.

Dupion. A fabric made from slub rayon threads and is used for curtains. (Slub threads have irregularities in their thickness.)

Felt. A fabric produced from densely matted (felted) wool. It is used under table cloths, and as carpet underlays when it can be impregnated with latex.

Fibre glass. A fabric woven from fine filaments of glass which is fireproof. It is used for light-weight curtains and shower curtains and should only be washed by hand.

Flame resistant fabrics. Pure wool, glass fibre and asbestos fabrics are inherently flameproof. All cotton, linen and most rayon fabrics can usually be flameproofed provided they have not had a special finish. It may be possible to flameproof other fabrics and there are firms who test samples and report on their suitability for flameproofing.

Flannelette. A brushed (teased) cotton fabric which, because it is fluffy, is soft and picks up dust easily and so is used for dusters. Also because of its fluffiness it is warmer than ordinary cotton fabrics, and is sometimes used for sheets and underblankets. It must not be confused with flannel, which is a woollen fabric.

Folkweave. A loosely woven cotton fabric from coarse, coloured yarns used in simple designs, and often with textural or three-dimensional effects. It is used for curtains and bedspreads.

Gingham. A plain, woven fabric, normally of cotton, with a check or striped design. It is used for bathroom curtains and as dust sheets.

Hessian. A coarse, fawn coloured, plain woven fabric, usually of jute, and used for protective coverings, e.g. bed underlays and oven cloths. It may be dyed and used as a wall covering.

Huckaback. A linen or cotton fabric in a huckaback weave and used for face, hand and continuous roller towels.

Milium. A metallic fabric used as linings for curtains because of its insulating properties.

Moquette. A cut or uncut pile fabric, or a combination of the two forming a pattern. An all wool or mohair pile on a cotton ground is the best quality, but cotton and rayon piles are hardwearing. Its main use is for upholstery.

Net. A very open or meshed fabric in which the threads may be twisted, knotted or woven together. It is made from many fibres but especially terylene, and is used for glass (sheer) curtains.

Percale. A plain woven cotton fabric made from Egyptian cotton. It is used for bed linen and was first used in American hotels.

Plush. A cut pile fabric with a deeper pile than velvet, but less closely woven. It is made of cotton, silk, mohair or man-made fibre and is very durable. It is used for upholstery and curtains.

Ratiné. A fabric of plain or twill weave in which the warp is made of spiral threads or has knob-like irregularities, producing a rough texture. It is used for upholstery, curtains and loose covers.

Repp. A plain woven, coloured fabric with a marked rib running from selvedge to selvedge, formed by using a fine warp and a coarser weft. It is most often made of cotton but can be of silk or man-made fibres. It is hardwearing and is used for upholstery, curtains and loose covers.

Sateen. A cotton fabric of weft satin weave used for lining curtains, and for the underside of quilts as it is not as slippery as many fabrics chosen for the top.

Satin. A smooth, lustrous fabric woven in satin weave (warp faced). Originally it was of all silk, but now many fibres are used giving rayon satin, cotton satin, etc. It comes in a variety of weights and may be used for curtains, bedspreads and cushion covers.

Scrim. A loosely woven, plain weave linen used where a lint-free cloth is required for cleaning.

Seersucker. A fabric with a puckered or crinkled appearance, usually made of cotton or man-made fibres and used mainly for bedspreads.

Serge. A heavy fabric of twill weave, originally all wool but now blends of cotton and man-made fibres are used. It is very hardwearing and used for tailored uniforms.

Sheeting. A plain or twill woven fabric, produced in a variety of qualities and used for sheets.

Taffeta. A plain woven fabric with a slightly thicker weft than warp producing a very fine rib. Originally it was all silk but now more generally contains rayon or other man-made fibres. It is used for bedspreads and cushion covers.

Tapestry. A closely woven, patterned fabric in which the pattern is formed by coloured weft threads. Originally it was hand woven and all wool; now wool, cotton, rayon or mixtures are used and the name is given to many closely woven, patterned fabrics. It is used for upholstery and the lighter weights can be used for curtains and loose covers.

Textured fabrics. Fabrics made from coarse yarns in novelty weaves, used to give rough or three-dimensional textures.

Ticking. A closely woven fabric in twill or satin weave. It was originally striped, but now is more often patterned when covering mattresses and divan bases, or white when enclosing the filling for cushions and pillows.

Towelling. A reversible uncut cotton or linen pile fabric of turkish (terry) weave and used for towels and bathmats.

Tweed. A heavy woollen fabric in plain or twill weave used for upholstery and curtains.

Union. A fabric made of a mixture of threads, cotton/linen, wool/cotton, polyester/cotton, etc.

Velour. A cut, warp pile fabric in which the pile has a tendency to lie down. It is normally made of cotton and is sometimes called cotton velvet, but rayon is in some cases used. It is used for upholstery and curtains.

Velvet. A cut, warp pile fabric in which the pile is woven over wires and cut. It was originally all silk, but now cotton and many of the man-made fibres are used when it should be called cotton pile velvet, rayon pile velvet, etc. There is great variety in weight, and it is used for upholstery, curtains and cushions.

Velveteen. A cut, weft pile fabric. Originally it was all cotton, but today the pile may be of rayon or mercerised cotton to look more like velvet, and the pile is generally shorter than in velvet.

Wild silk. A fabric made from silk obtained from the silk worm of the wild moth. The filaments are irregular in thickness and produce slubs in the fabric which is hardwearing and is used for curtains and wall coverings.

6

Soft Furnishings

Soft furnishings include curtains, loose covers, cushions, bedspreads and quilts (but not carpets), and they contribute greatly to the appearance of the room by bringing to it colour, pattern and texture. Some articles give protection, and some, in addition, give warmth and comfort. As each is subjected to different types and amounts of wear and tear, it follows that the fabric from which it is made should be suitable for the purpose.

Curtains

Curtains are used to give privacy where windows may be overlooked, to darken the room when necessary, and to bring character and atmosphere to the room by their line, colour, pattern and texture.

Curtains are essential to the appearance of any window and almost any furnishing fabric can be used. However, the weight, colour and pattern of the fabric will be determined by the size and position of the window, and the general character of the room.

The fabric should be chosen in regard to its resistance to fading and abrasion, its drape and dimensional stability, its flame resistance and cleanability.

The fabric's life expectancy is related to its amount of exposure to sunlight and airborne soiling. Fibres such as glass fibre, terylene, acrylics, saran/viscose rayon blends and brightly coloured nylons withstand sunlight well. Yellowing due to fibre oxidation occurs mainly in cotton, linen and rayon fabrics. 'Colourfast' can be an ambiguous term as it does not necessarily mean that the colour is fast under all conditions of use. Fabrics lose their colour brilliancy by water spotting, dry cleaning and rubbing as well as by fading by sunlight.

Curtains are subjected to abrasion by being pulled, being brushed against, rubbing along the floor and rubbing against window frames and sills. Abrasion can take place as well during laundering and dry cleaning. The abrasion resistance of the fabric will depend on the fibre and the construction of the yarn and fabric. Nylon, and terylene have excellent abrasion resistant properties, wool, cotton, linen and high tenacity rayons wear well in this respect also. Silk has most of the properties required for curtains but it is very expensive so silk fabrics are only used in luxury establishments.

Curtains are required to drape well and hold their shape but loosely woven fabrics tend to drop unevenly and with constant hand drawing the sides of the curtains may go out of shape.

The ease with which a fabric burns depends on the fibre or blends of fibres from which it is made; pure wool, glass fibre, asbestos, saran blend and modacrylics are inherently flame proof. A fabric that is closely woven is less likely to burn than one that is loosely woven. If curtains are fire proofed they should be marked as fire proofing may be affected by laundering and make reproofing necessary.

Airborne soiling and acid can do great damage to the curtain fabric so there should be a regular and thorough maintenance programme.

Most curtains are laundered or dry cleaned when necessary but it is always best to have lined curtains dry cleaned and although dry cleaning is expensive the curtains last longer.

Curtains need to be suspended from a horizontal rod or traverse track which may be of metal, wood or plastic, and may be the width of the window or extend either side of the window frame. When the latter is the case the curtains can be drawn well back giving width to a narrow window, preventing fading of the folds of material nearest the window, and allowing more light to enter the room (see p. 200). A curved track can be obtained for use at a bow window. When pelmets or valances are used it is a good idea to have an overlap in the centre of the track so that curtains really meet. However, decorative headings to curtains are more usual in many places now and the more modern track or rod is better in appearance.

Curtains are fixed to the track by rings or hooks and drop to the floor, or to the window sill where architectural aspects dictate, i.e. the shape of the window, radiators, or fitted furniture beneath it. They are normally of some opaque material, with sufficient fullness so that they can be drawn across the window to give complete privacy, some heat and sound insulation and a good appearance.

There is a wide variety of fabrics suitable for ordinary curtaining, and the choice will depend on the type of establishment and the particular room for which it is required. Sometimes different curtains are provided for winter and summer use.

For public rooms, it is probably wise to buy as good a material as can be afforded, and such fabrics as armures, brocades, damasks, heavy satins, printed linens, tapestries, velvets, novelty weaves and many others are suitable in the right setting (see Chapter 5).

For bedrooms, a less heavy material can be used; it will probably be less expensive and more easily maintained. Printed cottons, chintz, damask, cotton and rayon satins, repps, cretonne and printed linens are some which may be chosen.

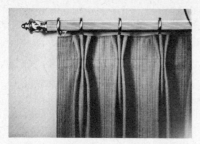

Pinch pleated curtain suspended from rod and rings

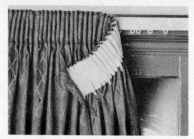

Pinch pleated curtain suspended from modern rail

In bathrooms, the windows are often of opaque glass when curtains are not necessary, except for appearance. If used, curtains are usually unlined and of some easily washed material. Nylon, plastic and glass fibre materials are sometimes used to curtain the showers, as these materials are non-absorbent and easily sponged of splash marks, but plastic material needs careful pulling because it goes stiff in time and with careless use tears occur. In some places curtains are found in rooms with no windows, e.g. lower ground floor banqueting rooms, and with careful use of fabric, lighting and air conditioning, the lack of windows may not be apparent. In some hotel bed-sitting rooms curtains are used to divide the bed area from the sitting area and in hospitals curtains separate beds (cubicles).

When choosing fabric for curtains it should always be seen in a large

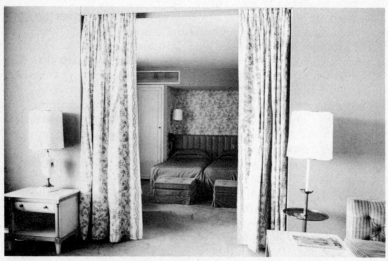

Curtains used as room dividers

piece, hanging in folds as the pattern quite frequently looks different when lying flat. It should be remembered that the light comes from behind the material during the day whereas at night it falls on the material. Materials with white backgrounds often lose their whiteness and fresh appearance after several cleanings, and so are best avoided. If a material has a large 'drop' in the pattern wastage may occur when matching up the curtains. Curtain mate-

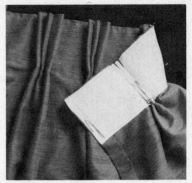

Pinch pleats showing reverse

rials may be 80 cm, 120 cm, 126 cm in width while some are much wider, and in order that the curtains hang well, the minimum width should be 1½ times the width of the rod or track.

Good curtains are usually lined and heavy curtains are often interlined. The lining enables the curtain to hang better, to be protected from dirt and sunlight, to give a uniform appearance from outside, and to afford greater insulation (i.e. keep heat in and cold out). The lining is often cream or beige sateen (or a colour which matches the background of the curtains) and is obtained in widths of 91 cm, 121 cm and 137 cm. A metallic fabric, milium, having good insulating properties is also being used as a lining material, and the interlining is the flannelette fabric 'bump'.

Curtains should never hang long without cleaning, as dust and soot rot the fabric. Because there are many curtains of varying lengths in any one establishment it saves endless trouble if they are marked for the various rooms.

General points to be remembered in connection with curtains:

1 Velvet and other pile fabrics should hang with the pile running downwards and they tend to hold dust and the smell of smoke.

2 15–30 cm, according to the type and weight of material, should be allowed for hem and turning on each curtain.

3 Curtains when floor length should be 1.5–2.5 cm above floor level to prevent friction.

4 The minimum width of any curtain should be 1½ times the width of the track, but for light-weight fabrics and certain curtain headings, twice or even more is necessary.

5 Curtain headings may be of various types, e.g. gathered or fix pleated, by the use of special tapes and the appropriate hooks or rings by which the curtain is attached to the rod or track.

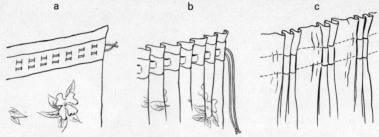

To show the use of special tapes for curtain headings

6 The lining should be fixed to the top and the sides of the curtain, but the hem should not be attached.

7 Hems and sides of good quality curtains should always be hand sewn and never machined.

8 Heavy curtains may have weights or even a chain in the hems to improve the hang.

9 Draw cords or rods may be used to facilitate the pulling of curtains and to prevent the marking of the fabric.

10 It is necessary to have curtains flame proofed in places where entertainment takes place.

Non-drawing curtains. In some circumstances curtains may be needed for decoration and are not made to draw, for example where there is an opening into an alcove, or with mock windows, or venetian blinds, etc. They are normally narrower than ordinary curtains and may be looped back at the side in various ways.

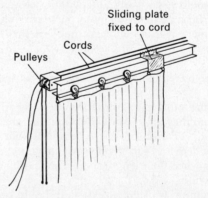

To show draw cords

Pelmets, valances, swags. Pelmets and valances are decorative headings fixed over the top of the curtain to hide the suspension, to add decoration to the room, and in some cases to alter the apparent size of the window.

Pelmets are rigid, and may be of shaped pieces of wood or hardboard which can be painted to match the décor of the room, or they may be of padded plastic or stiffened fabric to match or contrast with the curtains. The fabric is mounted on stiff buckram and is often tailored to fit the window.

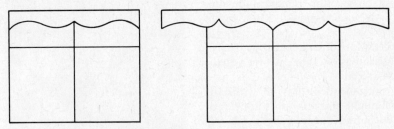

To show shaped pelmets and the effect of different length pelmets on the apparent size of a window

A valance is made of frilled or pleated material and fixed to a valance rail.

A swag is a draped finish to hide the curtain heading and is frequently completed with a tail.

Net curtains. Net, sheer or glass curtains are made of translucent fabrics, frequently terylene net, which soften and diffuse the light as it passes through them. The curtains are used where windows can be overlooked, and are placed close to the window where they hold some of the dirt which would otherwise get on to the main curtains. They are held by rod or stretched plastic coated wire through the top hem, and a drop rod is particularly useful for long net curtains, so that they can be lowered and changed easily without the use of a pair of steps.

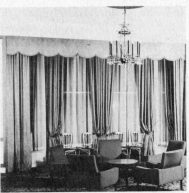

Curtains showing a pelmet

With these light-weight fabrics the curtains should be two to three times the width of the window, and there should be sufficient weight at the bottom of the curtains to enable them to hang properly. This can be achieved by using treble hems, and with casement windows it is a good idea to have a rod or stretched wire through the bottom as well as the top hem, to prevent the curtains blowing outside, but the curtains must not impede the opening of the window.

Net curtains become soiled very easily and require frequent changing, so it is essential that there are at least two sets per window. Where there are different sized windows, the curtains should be marked.

There is considerable choice of materials for net curtains, white or pale coloured, patterned or plain, made of cotton or man-made fibres. It is wise to buy the best quality possible, as crispness and translucency are often affected by frequent washings in the poorer quality materials. Terylene net, is to be recommended, as it withstands sunlight and retains its appearance after frequent washings. Unless the curtains are stretched and held in position top and bottom, terylene

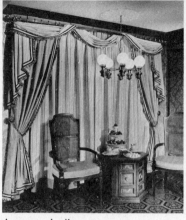

A swag and tail

net must be pressed after washing, with a warm iron.

Other fabrics for sheer curtains include a net curtaining with a metallic backing. Aluminium particles are bonded onto a polyester net when 45–65% of the sun's radiation may be reflected.

Aluminium or steel wire mesh in a variety of colours will drape and can be used as curtains or partition material, as can metal chain.

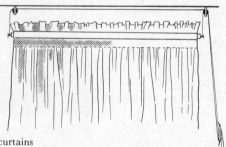

A 'drop rod' for net curtains

Care and cleaning of curtains

1 Keep rod and track free from dust by the use of a feather flick, a wall broom or a vacuum cleaner attachment.

2 Shake often. Use vacuum cleaner attachment or brush occasionally to remove dust from the curtains.

3 Deal appropriately with repairs to linings, frayed edges and any difficulties with pulling, bent tracks, etc.

4 Reverse the position of the curtains so that no part is continually exposed to the sun.

5 Have lined curtains dry cleaned; if unlined, and of a suitable material, have them laundered.

Blinds

Venetian blinds are sometimes used in place of net curtains where windows can be overlooked. In some cases, ordinary curtains may be dispensed with, and the venetian blinds used with side drapes or strip framing, when there may be a considerable saving in materials.

Venetian blinds require constant care and cleaning, cut off a great deal of light if attached to the window head, even when raised, and *guests* complain of their noise. Vertical slat blinds are also available.

Many blinds of the roller type are available and they may be gaily patterned. When used on their own they do not give the well finished appearance of a good curtained window but it is possible to use them with non-drawing curtains thus saving curtain material. If used to give privacy instead of net curtains they tend to obstruct the light but they are much easier to keep clean than venetian blinds as they are easily dusted and wiped over when necessary.

Care and cleaning

1   Attend to badly hanging blinds.
2   Dust or feather flick frequently.
3   Wash with warm water and synthetic detergent as often as required. This may be a contract job when they will normally be taken down and cleaned.

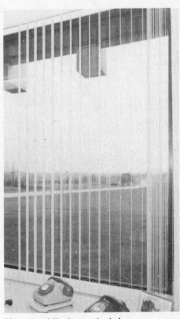

Venetian blinds: vertical slats

Loose Covers

Loose covers are detachable covers fitted over upholstered chairs, stools, etc. They can give a clean, fresh appearance to a room, but the constant need to straighten them and to keep them well maintained are reasons why some places no longer use them.

Loose covers may be used to cover shabbiness, to protect the original upholstery and to change the appearance of the room (e.g. winter and summer coverings). The covers may reach almost to floor level with a pleated or gathered 'skirt' or they may be tailored and fixed under the chair.

Fastenings may be hooks and eyes, zips or the 'touch and close' fasteners. The last consists of two nylon strips, one with thousands of tiny hooks and the other with thousands of tiny loops, and when pressed together the hooks grip the loops to give a light and secure closure, yet can be easily peeled apart. These fasteners can be washed or dry cleaned without damage.

Whereas almost any material can be used for curtains, closely woven fabrics are to be preferred for loose covers, e.g. chintz, cretonne, etc. These withstand abrasion, are less likely to snag, will not allow dust to filter through to the upholstery beneath, and will hold their shape better than loosely woven ones. A material which does not crease badly is an added advantage.

The choice of pattern, colour and texture is as for any other soft furnishing in that the material must be in keeping with the room and the rest of the furnishings. In some rooms, material matching the

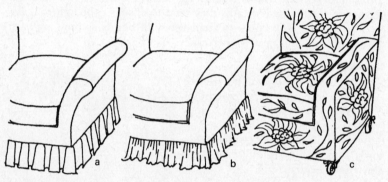

(a) a pleated skirt; (b) a frilled skirt and (c) a tailored cover with ties underneath

curtains is used, but normally this is better restricted to one or two pieces of furniture, or it may become too dominant and, if patterned, the room appear overpatterned. Loose covers are sometimes considered a cheap substitute for re-upholstering but in reality they may cost nearly as much.

Loose covers may be laundered, but many are better dry cleaned as they are liable to shrink when washed and great difficulty will be experienced when putting them on again. There are nylon stretch covers which are easily laundered, do not shrink and because of their 'stretch' are easy to put on but they may not be suitable for all shapes of chairs. All chairs and covers should be marked so that it can be seen to which chair a cover belongs.

To protect upholstered furniture from soiling in the most likely places, shields for arms and backs (antimacassars) are frequently used. These may be of matching material to the loose covers or of white or cream linen. They require to be washed frequently, and need to be fixed firmly to the chair by special pins or the touch and close fastening, or they present a very untidy appearance to the room.

Care and cleaning
1 Shake and tidy frequently.
2 Brush or vacuum clean regularly.
3 Attend to repairs.
4 Have laundered or dry cleaned as required.

Cushions

Cushions may be used to increase the comfort of chairs and couches and to bring colour, pattern and texture to the room. They require constant attention because they are often removed from their normal places, and feather ones all too easily become squashed and untidy looking and in need of repair.

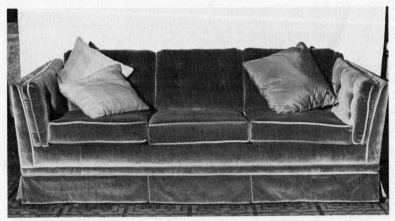

Fitted and scatter cushions

Cushions may be all shapes and sizes filled with down, feather or kapok and covered in a variety of materials, e.g. velvet or taffeta and often in gay colours with cord or fancy edgings. The covers may be fastened in a similar way to loose covers.

Care and cleaning
1 Shake and tidy frequently.
2 Repair when necessary.
3 Brush or vacuum regularly.
4 Remove covers and wash or dry clean them as required.

Bedspreads and quilts are dealt with in Chapter 10.

7

Floor Finishes

Floors are large important areas readily noticed on entering a room or particular area and they may be both functional and decorative. They play a very large part in the cleaning and maintenance programme of any establishment. They cover a tremendous area and are subjected to a great deal of wear and tear. In order that they should remain in an hygienic condition and retain as good an appearance for as long as is possible, some knowledge of the various types of floor finishes, their advantages, disadvantages and maintenance is necessary. Floors frequently form the basis on which the rest of the décor is planned, outlasting other furnishings and decorations and clean, well kept floor surfaces will often indicate the standard of cleanliness throughout the establishment.

It is essential that the floor finish chosen for any particular place should be in keeping with the purpose of the room. There may be places where durability and hygiene are of more importance than appearance, for instance in the kitchen; while on the other hand, appearance is of prime importance in the lounge where an impression of warmth, comfort and quietness is expected.

Floor finishes will only in rare cases be chosen solely for luxury and normally the following points should be given consideration:

1   The appearance requirements of the area

This may be one of luxury or utility and the flooring in some areas, more than in others, will be relied on to contribute to the aesthetic value of the room, when the material of the flooring, its colour and its pattern are of great importance.

The colour of the flooring and the amount of light reflected from it (depending on the shininess or dullness of the surface) can influence the atmosphere of the room. Pale colours, especially blues and greens as well as shiny surfaces, give a cool or cold appearance while other colours and a more matt surface give an impression of warmth.

The size of the pattern has a strong influence on the sense of scale in the room. Thus, patterned floorings tend to make a large room appear smaller and plain colours have the reverse effect making a small room seem larger.

Some colours and patterns retain their appearance of cleanliness longer than others by not showing so readily spillages and other soiling, e.g. dirty footprints and heelmarks.

2   The comfort requirements of the area

The comfort with which a flooring is walked on depends on whether the surface is hard or soft, resilient or 'dead'. While soft, resilient floorings are comfortable to walk on generally, they can prove extremely tiring to people, e.g. waiters in the restaurant, continually walking on them.

Softness, resilience, quietness and warmth properties of a flooring tend to go together, and the harder, noisier, colder floorings offer less heat and sound insulation. A noisy flooring may cause disturbance, hence discomfort, to the occupants of the room and to those in adjacent rooms. Some floorings tend to be more slippery than others and this, too, may lead to discomfort, although slipperiness may not always be due to the flooring itself but due to the maintenance given to the flooring once it has been laid.

3   The wear and tear expectancy of the area

The type and amount of traffic will vary from place to place. In areas where this has not been considered sufficiently before a flooring has been chosen, the flooring may become shabby looking very quickly and the tone of the establishment brought down by the 'tired' looking floor. (The same thing can happen with faulty maintenance.)

Some areas more than others will have much more grit and moisture brought on to them from outside. Grit is a great enemy of any flooring, but some will stand up to it better than others. Spillages of water, grease and food acids are likely to occur more frequently in some places and may harm certain floorings. Cigarette burns, the dragging of furniture and the use of trolleys are other possibilities which must not be forgotten.

There are, too, areas of more concentrated wear, for example the foyer or entrance hall where large numbers of people walk (apart from generally more traffic, traffic lanes to the reception desk, enquiry desk, lift, etc., may show) also room entrances from the corridor. The flooring at the bar, at the dressing table, at waiters' stations and other places where the feet are ground into the flooring as people turn, may all show excessive wear.

4   The ease of cleaning in relation to the type and amount of soiling expected

The cleaning of floors is an important item in the running costs of any establishment and it is possible that the extra initial cost which may be

involved in providing a flooring which is easier to maintain will be
saved over a comparatively short time—of course, there must be the
capital available for the extra initial cost.

It is the flooring material which determines the ease of cleaning, but
it should be realised that because a flooring is easy to clean it does not
necessarily retain a clean appearance throughout the day. Floorings are
constantly being soiled, but they cannot usually be constantly cleaned
(however easy it is). Some floorings keep their appearance of cleanliness
better than others when, in fact, they are heavily soiled; this depends
not only on the flooring material but also on the colour and pattern
chosen.

5   The length of life expected from the flooring

The flooring of a kitchen, hospital ward, basement corridor, etc., may
be expected to last for many years but, owing to changes in décor a
bedroom flooring may not be expected to have more than seven or eight
years' life or a bar flooring more than two or three years, especially if
it is of a contemporary nature. Thus the flooring needs to be durable
under the conditions of use, for the length of life expected, and in conse-
quence it is not always necessary to buy the most durable or the most
expensive material.

6   The money available

This may limit the choice of flooring and is always an important
consideration. The true cost of a flooring is the initial cost including
laying plus estimated maintenance cost. (In certain hospitals it has been
estimated that the cost to maintain a corridor ranged between £40–£65
per 92.9 m^2 (1000 sq. ft.) per year.)

The effective life of most floorings will depend on how they were laid
initially and on their subsequent care and cleaning. Many properties
of a flooring may be enhanced or ruined by the base, i.e. the subfloor,
on which the flooring is laid.

In large modern buildings the subfloor is often made of concrete, but
in older and smaller buildings it consists of soft wood boards, at least
10 cm wide nailed to wooden joists.

Softwoods are obtained from the cone bearing trees, e.g. European
Redwood (Deal), Spruce, Douglas fir, Pitchpine, and Deal is the most
frequently used soft wood for these boards; it is poor in appearance and
not very hardwearing. It is seldom left white and uncovered these days,
owing to the need for scrubbing and the consequent harmful effect of
the water on the wood. Where such a floor is only partially covered with
a carpet, the boards may, however, be stained and varnished and left
as a surround, but they are more usually completely covered with a floor

finish. Even with careful seasoning or kiln drying, these boards often warp and shrink leaving gaps through which draughts and dust will rise. The shrinkage, which may be due to central heating, also causes the boards to creak and squeak and this can be a source of annoyance which requires attention. These wooden subfloors must be adequately ventilated to prevent the growth of fungi, producing dry rot, and this is one of the reasons that air bricks are introduced into the walls of the building.

Concrete subfloors have the advantage of being solid, allowing the use of underfloor heating, and not creaking or requiring ventilation. There is, however, a risk of rising damp when they are placed in direct contact with the ground, and a screed of suitable material should be applied before many of the floor finishes. Ordinary concrete floors are dusty and difficult to clean, and where they have to be left uncovered they should be treated with a dust preventative, e.g. sodium silicate. Aerated concrete is available to increase sound and heat insulation.

A flooring should be provided with a true, level and dry subfloor. Where the finish is in tile form, the tiles should be laid evenly and close together, so preventing dirt and bacteria accumulating in the crevices. This type of flooring has the advantage that individual tiles which have become worn or damaged can be replaced. A floor finish laid *in situ* normally presents a jointless flooring and may for easier cleaning be continued up the wall to give a coved skirting.

Once a floor finish or flooring is laid, the treatment given to it is of tremendous importance, in order to prevent the penetration of dirt and to provide an easily maintained surface. It is for these reasons that many floorings today are sealed and/or polished.

A seal is applied to a clean, dry floor and gives a non-absorbent, semi-permanent gloss or finish which will wear in time. Before the floor can be re-sealed, any remaining seal has normally to be stripped off, and this can be done in the case of wood and cork floorings by sanding, but in other cases a chemical stripper generally has to be used. These chemicals are fairly drastic in their action, and before using a seal the reaction of the flooring to the stripper should be considered. In order to preserve the seal for as long as possible a polish may be applied to sealed floorings. Polishes are also applied to unsealed floorings when they prevent the penetration of dirt.

Floor finishes are, in general, harmed by either spirit or water and the choice of polish rests on this fact, as polishes are either spirit or water based. Spirit based floor polishes may be paste or liquid and require buffing when dry to produce a shine; water based polishes which may be water/wax or plastic emulsions are liquid, and dry to a shiny surface which in some cases can be improved by buffing, and in others cannot. It is this ability to dry shiny that has confused water based or self-shining emulsion polishes with floor seals (see p. 36).

The amount of cleaning required by any flooring will depend largely on the amount and type of traffic it receives, but some form of daily cleaning will be necessary, while special cleaning will be required at less frequent intervals.

Daily cleaning entails the removal of

(a) dust and dirt by sweeping, mopping, vacuum cleaning, damp mopping or washing according to the type of flooring, and when washing, excess water should be avoided. While a flooring material may be unharmed by water, the adhesive used with it may be damaged and cause the lifting of the flooring, particularly if in tile form.

(b) resistant marks, normally by rubbing with a damp cloth and a little fine scouring powder.

(c) stains which should be removed as soon as possible, as on drying they become set and are much more difficult to remove.

Special cleaning methods are given in the chart on p. 142.

To prevent accidents and further damage to the flooring

(a) Loose edges should be attended to immediately.

(b) Metal strips should be placed over the edge of the flooring at doorways, staircases, etc.

(c) Spillages should be wiped up as soon as possible.

(d) Excess water and polish should be avoided during cleaning.

Having decided what requirements are to be met by the floor finish, it is possible to consider the types of finishes which may suit the particular area and a choice may be made from the following:

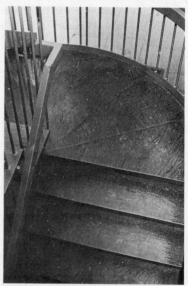

Granolithic, terrazzo and other cementitious finishes laid *in situ* or in tile form.

Stone—marble, slate etc. in slab form.

Magnesite and other composition finishes laid *in situ* or in the form of small blocks.

Bitumastic finishes laid *in situ*.

Ceramic tiled floorings—quarries and more decorative, highly glazed tiles.

Epoxy, polyester and polyurethane resin seamless finishes.

Wood—hardwoods laid as strip, block or parquet.

Thermoplastic tiled floorings.

Vinyl floorings in tile or sheet form.

Rubber floorings in tile or sheet form.

A slate staircase

Linoleum in tile or sheet form.

Cork in tile or sheet form.

Carpets are normally regarded as floor coverings rather than floor finishes.

Hard Finishes

Hard finishes are, in general, durable, noisy, and cold in appearance. Most are vermin proof, impervious to dry rot, fire resistant and easily cleaned and where laid *in situ* they may have coved edges to facilitate cleaning.

Granolithic

Granolithic is a hard floor finish of graded granite chips set in cement, as against concrete which is sand and cement. It is laid in a plastic state on a solid subfloor, and should continue 2.5–5 cm up the wall to form a curved edge or coved skirting which makes cleaning easier. Half channel drainage pipes connected to a trapped gulley may be incorporated when a slight slope to the drainage outlet will facilitate scrubbing and swilling of the floor surface. Pre-cast slabs with lifting rings and set in brass surrounds, may be used to cover drains and other service pipes to render them accessible.

Granolithic is a heavy-duty floor and is used for basement corridors, store rooms, stairways and laundries. It can, however, be brought to a smooth surface by machine grinding when it has a more decorative appearance and may be used in cloakrooms, corridors and kitchens.

Terrazzo

Terrazzo is also a hard floor finish, consisting of a mixture of marble and other decorative chips or pieces, set in a fine cement which can be coloured. The floor is machine ground to give a smooth surface and is extremely durable.

Marble is a special form of rock mainly found in Italy, and may be white, black, green or brown in colour, and when used for floorings is normally laid in slab form, and is very expensive although a cheaper form, travertine marble, is also used. Travertine marble has small cavities in it which offer some slip resistance but which are sometimes filled with cement. Terrazzo being only of small pieces of marble is much cheaper. It is laid *in situ* or as pre-cast tiles when the marble pieces may be up to 10 cm in size. For an *in situ* flooring the marble is much smaller and coved skirtings can be made or it may continue up the wall as a dado. Where the floor area to be covered is large the terrazzo is normally divided into sections by means of brass or ebonite strips to allow for

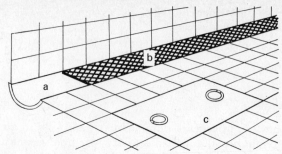

(a) half channel drainage pipe with
(b) metal covering,
(c) a precast slab with lifting rings

slight expansion and originally thought to help control cracking but now used more for decoration.

Terrazzo can be an attractive flooring if well maintained and its variegated pattern can camouflage dust and dirt to some extent. Cement is absorbent and strong alkalis should be avoided in cleaning as the high percentage of dissolved solids, e.g. soda, may lead to crystals being left in the matrix after evaporation of the water and these exert pressure and may cause the surface to crack. Marble is susceptible to attack by acids when pitting may result.

Terrazzo and granolithic floorings have the usual properties of hard floorings and can have a drain incorporated.

Due to its absorbent nature terrazzo flooring may be marked by oil and spillages such as ink, beverages, etc. Its smoothness may present a slippery surface and when used on a staircase a non-slip nosing is necessary. It is also used in entrance halls and cloakrooms. Terrazzo is liable to crack if not in tile form. As near neutral a detergent as possible should be used in cleaning as terrazzo is affected by acids and strong alkalis. In male cloakrooms stains around the urinals may give problems. (see chart on p. 143 for cleaning).

Other stones used as floorings are sandstone, quartzite and slate. They are all hard wearing and obtainable in a variety of colours. Sawn or polished finishes tend to be slippery but riven finishes are non-slip.

Magnesite Oxychloride

Magnesite flooring consists of wood flour and other fillers mixed with burnt magnesite, and laid *in situ* or in the form of small blocks. This finish is extremely porous and washing should be avoided whenever possible. It is therefore used where there is little risk of water being spilt, e.g. linen rooms. It may be sealed and/or polished to prevent the penetration of water and dirt, but is then very slippery. Magnesite flooring is moderately warm in appearance and the initial cost is low but it is limited in colour and extremely porous. It is harmed by water, most chemicals and coarse abrasives (see chart on p. 143 for cleaning).

Bitumastic

Bitumastic flooring is a jointless flooring and consists of a type of asphalt rolled on to a solid subfloor in a hot plastic state when a sluice hole may be incorporated, and it can be continued up the wall as a coved skirting. It is soft in texture although its appearance is hard and it is completely impermeable to water. It is normally black, red or brown, but may have other colours rolled in, giving a mottled effect, or the surface may be painted. It is used in public bathrooms, in hospital corridors and to protect other floor finishes from rising damp when it is used as a damp-proof membrane.

Bitumastic flooring dents with heavy weights and softens with heat, is harmed by spirit, oil and acids but the initial cost is low (see chart on p. 142 for cleaning).

Ceramic tiles

Ceramics are clayware and the floor tiles are available in a great variety of qualities, colours and sizes.

Quarry tiles are made from a natural type of clay, often of several blends, and are fired under pressure to make them hard and durable. Different qualities are produced, and the harder tiles are less absorbent but more slippery; however, it is possible to obtain tiles with slightly abrasive surfaces so rendering them less slippery. The heather brown quarries are the most durable. The tiles may be of various thicknesses and are generally 10 cm, 15 cm or 23 cm square and red, yellow, buff or blue in colour. They should be laid close together on flat, even concrete in cement mortar and then grouted to seal the joints. This prevents dirt and bacteria accumulating in the crevices. Coved tiles and removable pre-cast slabs (to cover service pipes) are available to facilitate cleaning and maintenance. When laid properly quarry tiles form an impervious, hard wearing surface and are used in cloakrooms, kitchens, canteens and any place used for the preparation or storage of food.

Ceramic tiles with a particularly hard glaze, are used as more decorative floorings. There is a very much wider range of colours and they are often used in bathrooms of the more luxurious type, patios and similar places in colours harmonising with the wall tiles. Tessellated tiles are small ceramic tiles often used as mosaics, giving a highly decorative floor.

Ceramic tiles are not affected by water, grease, acids or alkalis but the grouting may be, and so strong alkaline cleansers should be avoided. They may crack or break with heavy weights and marks can be difficult to remove if left. The initial cost may be high but this must be offset by the need for little upkeep (see chart on p. 142 for cleaning).

Resin seamless floorings

Synthetic resins with appropriate hardeners or curing agents may be poured or trowelled on to a floor to give an easily cleaned, hygienic, jointless floor finish with coved edges. The resins used may be epoxy, polyester or polyurethane. Of the three, polyurethanes are the newest but have shown the greatest rate of increase in use. They are more resilient than epoxy or polyester floorings and are therefore quieter.

Decorative polyurethane floorings with vinyl chips or flakes, or marble chips embedded in the resin, are available and there is a wide range of colours and designs from which to choose. The final coats of polyurethane resin determine the exact finish and wear resistance. They may be carried up the wall as a covering.

They are extremely hard wearing, unaffected by spillages of water, food, alcohol and most chemicals. Due to the resilience of the resin the floorings show a good recovery to point load and in spite of the shiny surface they are non-skid.

Polyurethane floor finishes may be used in kitchens, canteens and other areas where food is handled, bathrooms, cloakrooms, corridors and laundries (see chart on p. 143 for cleaning).

Wood

Wood finishes of good quality are among the most beautiful floorings, providing the variety of the wood and the size of the unit are chosen for effect. These floorings, which are to be mainly uncovered and subjected to a good deal of wear, must be of hard woods which come from broad-leafed trees such as oak, teak, maple, walnut, birch, beech, etc. There are varying degrees of hardness and on the whole they give better resistance to abrasive wear and indentations than soft woods. (Pitchpine, a soft wood, is however, harder than some hardwoods, e.g. Agba, African walnut.) The choice of the individual species will vary according to its colour, the scale and definition of its grain, and its rate of wear. Rhodesian Teak, Muhimbi, East African Olive, Rock Maple, Missanda, Birch and Jarrah are exceptionally hard wearing woods. The first three are the more decorative. Birch, Maple and Jarrah are very suitable for ballroom floors.

The right choice of timber is very important as apart from grooves and splintering caused by bad wear, the opening up of joints may occur from wrong selection. To ensure close joints, attention must be paid to the moisture content of the timber at the time of laying. As wood is absorbent, the required minimum moisture content will depend on the degree of heating in the building, e.g. with intermittent heating 12–16 per cent.; with central heating 10–14 per cent.

To prevent absorption of spills and dirt, wood floorings should be sealed and/or polished when any 'build-up' of polish should be avoided. Before polishing the flooring should be free from dust and dirt. Water is harmful to wood floorings, especially if they are unsealed, and strong alkalis cause wood to disintegrate, discolour and splinter. Wood floorings can be renovated by sanding with comparative ease after excessive wear or neglect, so that a new surface is exposed.

Strip wood flooring. A strip wood flooring consists of lengths of narrow strips (under 10 cm wide) of hardwood of good appearance, e.g. maple. The boards are fixed to joists or to timber insets in concrete, and this construction, together with the length of the strips, gives the floor its resilience and makes it very suitable for ballroom floors. A sprung floor has springs under the joists to increase the resilience.

Wood block flooring. A wood block flooring may be of two kinds, either (a) rectangular blocks (23 x 7.6 cm or 30 x 5 cm and 2.5–5 cm thick) generally laid in a herringbone pattern, or (b) smaller blocks often laid in basket pattern as a mosaic and made into panels for easy laying. The panels may be 45 cm square and faced with paper or backed with felt or aluminium according to manufacture.

Both types are laid in an adhesive on a level concrete base and made from woods of good appearance and durability, e.g. oak, teak, etc. and may be used in entrance halls and similar places where appearance is of importance.

The larger floor blocks are also used as a more utilitarian flooring when the woods will be chosen more for their durability than for their appearance e.g. Missanda, and may be found in linen rooms, storerooms and some offices.

Parquet flooring. Parquet flooring in appearance resembles a wood block flooring in that it also consists of rectangular pieces of wood (23 cm x 7.6 cm or 30 cm x 5 cm). However, it is manufactured from specially selected and kiln dried oak, walnut, teak and other decorative hardwoods. The blocks are very much thinner (less than 1 cm thick), and are pinned and glued to a wooden subfloor often in a herringbone pattern. Parquet is used in foyers and lounges in conjuction with rugs. A cheaper parquet flooring may have only a veneer of good quality wood on the surface and so forms a much less hard wearing floor.

Temporary wooden floorings, consisting of movable panels, may be laid on carpeted areas for dancing.

Wood floor finishes have a good appearance if well maintained and are poor conductors of heat and so are good insulators. Wood is resilient and wood floorings are therefore less tiring to walk on than unyielding substances. They are, however, inflammable and susceptible to dry rot; they become scratched and will splinter with the dragging of heavy articles. The initial cost is comparatively high, but if properly cared for the wood will mature and improve with age long after other materials have lost their appearance (see chart on p. 143 for cleaning).

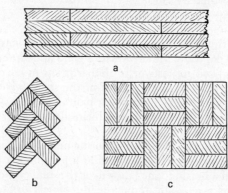

(a) strip wood flooring
(b) herringbone
(c) basket pattern

Semi-hard Finishes

Semi-hard finishes, sometimes called smooth floorings, are in general smooth, durable, resilient, of quite good appearance and relatively easily cleaned. Most of them are obtainable in sheet or tile form. There is a very wide range of price, colour and porosity although liquids can in most cases be easily removed from their surfaces. Care has to be taken in the choice of polish as some finishes are harmed by spirit and the porous ones by water.

Thermoplastic floor finishes

Thermoplastic floor tiles are made from a variety of asphaltic binders with inert fillers and pigments. They are rigid tiles, usually 23 cm square, and are laid on a clean, smooth, rigid surface, set as closely together as possible in an approved adhesive. They are laid in a warm, pliable state (thermoplastic) but harden on cooling and may be carried up the wall to form a small coved skirting. They may be polished with a water based polish, but polishing is liable to make them slippery.

They tend to be cold in appearance and because they have no resilience they are hard and noisy, dent with heavy weights and scratch easily, i.e. with grit, sharp edges, coarse abrasives. As they are thermoplastic they soften with heat and they will then dent more easily.

Thermoplastic tiles are non-porous, but strong alkalis will remove their surface, rendering them porous; they are also harmed by grease and spirit. Although cleaning is relatively easy they show marks badly, e.g. heel marks.

They are durable, obtainable in a variety of colours and are a cheap flooring. Their use is normally where a greaseproof surface is not required and the initial cost is an important factor. They may be used in bathrooms, corridors, offices, etc. (see chart on p. 143 for cleaning).

Vinylised thermoplastic tiles are now available. The introduction of the vinyl resins greatly improves the colour and wearing qualities of the tile without increasing the price very much.

Vinyl floorings

Vinyl floor finishes are manufactured from PVC and similar synthetic resins, inert fillers and pigments. They are very much more resistant to damage than other semi-hard floorings, but discarded cigarette ends do scar the surface.

There are two main types:

1 *Vinyl asbestos* which is obtainable only in tile form. The fillers include short fibred asbestos. The tiles are rigid and similar in appearance and feel to thermoplastic tiles and are stuck to the subfloor with a suitable adhesive.

2 *Flexible vinyl* flooring which is obtainable in tile or sheet form. During manufacture plasticisers are added to render the product flexible and the sheets can be welded to form a completely impervious floor. Sometimes the basic mixture is mounted on canvas or some other suitable backing material, e.g. felt, foam rubber or cork, and these backing materials add to the resilience and softness of the flooring and contribute to the reduction of noise but even without these backing materials it is more comfortable underfoot than either of the two previously mentioned tile floorings. This type of flooring may or may not be stuck down.

The vinyl content of the flooring may be a surface layer only and a wear surface of about 0.5 mm is considered suitable for contract work. The homogeneous sheet or tile vinyl floorings are more expensive, but not necessarily superior to the floorings with a surface layer of vinyl. There is a type of flooring in which coloured PVC chips are embedded in tough transparent vinyl.

The greater the amount of vinyl in the flooring the greater the resistance to wear, grease, scratching and indentation to point load. Some are remarkably resistant to indentation. Owing to the almost impervious nature of the flooring very little polish, if any, is required.

Cushioned vinyl floorings are now available which contain a layer of foamed vinyl. These prove effective sound insulators and are more resilient than the other vinyl floorings. It is possible to produce textured effects when wood block, ceramic tile, rushmatting and even carpet may be simulated.

Vinyl floorings can be used in a great variety of places including bathrooms, corridors, canteens, offices, study bedrooms, hospital wards, etc., (see chart on p. 143 for cleaning).

Rubber

Rubber floorings are obtainable in tile and sheet form. During manufacture, rubber with filling materials and pigments is vulcanised (heated out of contact with air) to give a hard finish, and the resulting tiles or sheets may be of many colours. They should be laid in a suitable adhesive on a smooth subfloor, and may be left unprotected or polished with a water based polish.

Rubber flooring is soft, quiet, resilient and comfortable to walk on. It is extremely durable if properly maintained and a life of 20–30 years is not uncommon. It is non-absorbent and resists water. It is harmed by spirit, grease, sunlight, alkalis and coarse abrasives and it marks badly, especially with rubber heels. Polishing with a water based emulsion affords some protection against sunlight and the scuffing of rubber heels. Rubber flooring may be used in bars, entrance halls, canteens, etc.

Oil and grease resistant rubber tiles are now available (made from nitrile rubber) but the colour range is more limited.

Rubber can be used for an infinite variety of mats and mattings found in places where protection is required for the floor beneath. Front door mats, mats in front of service lifts, and nosings on stairs may therefore be made of rubber (see chart on p. 143 for cleaning).

Linoleum

Linoleum consists of a mixture of powdered cork, resin, linseed oil and pigments, put on a foundation of jute canvas and subjected to heat and pressure. The product is passed through polishing rollers and further treatment is given to harden it. It is possible to obtain factory-sealed linoleum which helps overcome the necessity for preparing and sealing ordinary linoleum. These difficulties occur particularly in areas in constant use.

The thickness to which the mixture is laid on the backing varies with the quality from 1.2–6.7 mm and 3.2–4.5 mm is most popular for such places as restaurants, bars, canteens and most contract usage. In good quality linoleum the colour and pattern are inlaid, i.e. right through to the backing, whereas in cheap qualities they may only be printed on the surface, and so wear off. Linoleum may be bought in rolls usually 182 cm wide, or in tiles. The tiles are always stuck down while the rolls may be stuck or laid loosely. In sheet form linoleum is liable to shrink, and unless stuck down the edges should overlap and be trimmed later.

Linoleum is reasonably priced and extremely hard wearing (there are places where it has been down 30–40 years). It is subject to denting and scratching, but there is a special toughened form available which does not dent or scratch so easily. It is absorbent unless sealed and only minimum amounts of water should be used when cleaning. Linoleum is harmed by coarse abrasives, alkalis and becomes slippery if over-polished. It is marked by cigarette ends and rubber heels, but the marks may be removed by light rubbing with fine steel wool, fine scouring powder or a paraffined rag. Linoleum may be sealed and/or polished and is used in many places, for example, linen rooms, hostel bedrooms, offices, corridors, bathrooms, canteens, hospital wards (see chart on p. 143 for cleaning).

Cork

Cork tiles are made from granulated cork, moulded into blocks which are subjected to pressure and high temperature. During this process the natural resins bind the granules, and the blocks are then cut into tiles of the required size and the required thickness, usually 0.5–1 cm. Variations in the brown colour of the tiles result from the different amounts of pressure and heat to which the blocks are subjected. Owing to their absorbent nature they are normally sealed and/or polished.

There are cork tiles covered with a vinyl surface and these have the resilience of cork and durability of vinyl. They are more expensive than ordinary cork tiles.

Cork floorings have a warm and restful appearance; they are quiet and can be sanded down to expose a new surface. They are absorbent, burnt by cigarette ends and have little resistance to indentation when granules may become loosened and lost.

Cork tiles can be used in offices, corridors, bathrooms when vinyl surfaced and as surrounds to carpets (see chart on p. 142 for cleaning.)

It has been stated that when choosing a floor finish for any given situation appearance, comfort, durability, ease of cleaning and the cost of the material (including laying) have to be taken into consideration.

It is not easy to compare the appearance of different finishes in the same way that comfort and durability can be compared, because there are variables which may affect the appearance of the same basic mate-

CLEANING OF FLOORINGS

Type of flooring	Special remarks	Daily clean	Special clean
Bitumastic	Avoid use of white spirit and paraffin Surface can be painted	Sweep, wash, mop or use electric scrubber with hot water and a synthetic detergent	As daily clean
Ceramic tiles		As above	As above Quarries–remove stubborn marks with steel wool or fine scouring powder
Cork	Avoid use of excess water and alkalis Should be sealed and/or polished as it is very absorbent. Can be sanded down *Sealed*: Reseal as required. May be polished using water based polish. Remove build up as necessary using hot water and special removal agent *Unsealed*: Polish with spirit based polish. Remove build up as necessary using white spirit and fine steel wool or nylon web pad. Rinse and re-wax. Can be sanded	*Sealed*: sweep, damp mop or vacuum clean *Unsealed and polished*: sweep, mop or vacuum clean. Buff with electric polisher	*Sealed*: if polished, repolish, spray buff or spray clean *Unsealed and polished*: re-wax using little polish and much buffing
Granolithic	Can be brought to a smooth finish by machine, to improve its appearance	As bitumastic	As bitumastic

Type of flooring	Special remarks	Daily clean	Special clean
Linoleum	Avoid scrubbing, coarse abrasives and alkalis *Sealed*: re-seal as required *Sealed and unsealed*: Polish using water based polish. Remove build up as necessary, using hot water and special removal agent	Sweep, mop or vacuum clean	Wash by hand or mop with hot water (used sparingly) and detergent If polished, repolish, spray buff or spray clean
Magnesite	Avoid use of water, alkalis, acids and coarse abrasives	Sweep, mop or vacuum clean	
Resin seamless		As ceramic tiles	As daily clean
Rubber	Avoid use of alkalis, spirits and coarse abrasives Use water based polish as linoleum	Sweep or damp mop	As linoleum
Terrazzo	Avoid use of acids and strong alkalis	As bitumastic	As daily clean Remove stubborn marks with fine scouring powder
Thermoplastic	As Rubber	As Rubber	As Rubber
Vinyl	As Rubber	As Rubber	As Rubber
Wood	As Cork	As Cork	As Cork

N.B. Sweeping with a broom should be avoided when possible. The use of a mop sweeper or vacuum cleaner is preferable.

Flooring	Approx. price range per square metre	Warmth to touch	Quietness (impact noise)	Resistance to			
				Slip	Wear	Water	Indentation
Hard							
Bitumastic	£2–£2·50	F	F	G–F	VG	VG	F–P
Ceramic tiles							
Quarries	£4–£20	VP	VP	G–F	VG	VG	VG
Hard glazed	£4–£15	VP	VP	G–F	VG	VG	VG
Granolithic	£1·50–£2·50	VP	VP	G–VP	VG–F	G	VG
Terrazzo	£5–£11	F	F	G–F	G	VP	VG–G
Marble	£11–£20	F	F	G	G–F	VG	VG
Magnesite	£2–£4	G	P	G–F	VG–F	P	G–F
Polyurethane resin	£2·50–£3·50	G	P	G–F	VG–F	P	G–F
Hard wood:							
oak strip	£6–£8	G	P	G–F	VG–F	P	G–F
oak block	£7–£9	G	P	G–F	VG–F	P	G–F
oak parquet	£10–£12	G	P	G–F	VG–F	P	G–F
Semi-hard							
Cork tiles	£2·50–£3	VG	VG	VG	G–F	VP	VP
Linoleum	£2–£3	G–F	G–F	G–F	G	F	P
Rubber	£2·50–£3·50	G–F	VG–G	G	VG–G	G	G–F
Thermoplastic	£1·75–£2·50	F–P	P	G–F	F	G	P
Vinyl asbestos	£1·75–£2·50	F–P	P	G–F	G	G	F
Vinyl flexible	£2·50–£5	G–F	G	G–F	VG–F	VG–F	G–F

VG = very good
G = good
F = fair
P = poor
VP = very poor

rial. The colour, pattern and texture all affect the appearance of the same flooring as well as its component shape, e.g. the size and shape of ceramic tiles.

Opposite is a table of some of the properties of the different types of floor finishes which can be more easily compared.

8

Carpets

Carpets are being used extensively nowadays in all types of establishments, as apart from their appearance, safety factor, warmth and sound insulation a very important advantage is their saving in cleaning costs.

Semi-hard floorings, e.g. linoleum, vinyl, etc., are cheaper than carpet initially, but demand daily sweeping or mopping, and buffing, with periodic stripping and re-waxing all of which are expensive in terms of time, labour, equipment and materials. In one investigation the cleaning cost of carpet was found to be 9/16 of that of the semi-hard floorings and so the higher initial cost of carpeting can be offset by the lower cleaning costs. In places where there are large carpeted areas the initial cost of the carpet may be completely paid for within its lifetime. Besides these direct savings in connection with carpeting there are others more indirect, such as reduced heating costs and economies in building costs.

Carpets originated in the East and were all hand made; now they are mainly machine made and in some cases may be reproductions of the original Eastern ones. There are many carpets from which to choose, with a wide price range and they may be laid on any dry, clean, smooth floor.

In general carpets consist of a backing or foundation and a surface pile which may be cut or uncut. A soundly constructed, firm backing is essential and this is normally made from jute or cotton threads, though others, e.g. linen, hemp, are also used. The pile yarn may be from wool, cotton, rayon, nylon, terylene, acrilan, courtelle, polypropylene, etc., and it is, of course, the basic element in the quality of the carpet. No fibre is perfect and so blends have become popular.

Wool because of its resilience and durability has been the main fibre used for many years. It is warm, does not soil or ignite readily and retains its appearance well if properly maintained. Nylon has excellent wearing qualities, dries quickly, stands up to salt and sand brought in on the shoes from icy roads and beaches, but does not compare with wool in regard to resilience or soil resistance and so a 100 per cent. nylon carpet does not retain its appearance as well as a 100 per cent. wool carpet. In addition nylon melts, e.g. with cigarette ends, and is electrostatic in dry conditions. Nowadays 80/20 per cent. wool/nylon blends are very popular when the main characteristics of wool will be retained, the abrasion resistance or wear quality of the carpet improved and a cheaper carpet made available.

The acrylics, acrilan and courtelle, resemble wool in handle and appearance more than nylon. Acrilan has good durability, resilience, and dyes more easily than other synthetic fibres. It does, however, melt. It is used as 100 per cent. whereas courtelle is used in blends. Courtelle takes a high twist which makes the carpets more resistant to shading and tracking. Terylene and polypropylene have good abrasion resistance but poor recovery from crushing; for this reason terylene with its soft handle is very suitable for the longer piled rugs and polypropylene for the bonded cloths.

Cotton has little resilience and fades badly and is not used for contract carpets. Rayon too has little resilience and its general properties do not compare with wool or the synthetics. It is, however, a cheaper fibre and when introduced into a blend, reduces the cost of the carpet considerably. (The cost of rayon is less than half the cost of other fibres used.) Evlan, a modified rayon, has improved properties and is now more frequently used in the blends.

Some of the blends besides 80/20 Wool/Nylon are

40% Courtelle/40% Evlan/20% Nylon

42½% Wool/42½% Evlan/15% Nylon

50% Courtelle/50% Evlan

The type of pile is extremely important as most of the wear falls on it, but without a good backing a hardwearing pile is insufficient for a good carpet. The quality of a carpet is dependent on the type of fibre or fibres used in it, as well as the closeness (there may be 125 tufts per sq. inch or 20 tufts per sq. cm), depth and firm anchorage of the pile. Each carpet must be judged for itself and not according to the method of manufacture as was previously thought possible.

Carpets may be woven, tufted or adhesively bonded according to their method of manufacture. It is possible in some countries, e.g. Holland, to obtain knitted carpets where a tight loop pile is knitted into the backing; the great advantage of knitted carpets is their speed of manufacture thus making them less expensive.

In woven carpets the backing and pile are produced together during the weaving process and different weaves are used to give the different types of carpets. Wilton and Axminster are the two woven carpets most frequently bought; these have a cut pile and until recently were made almost entirely of wool.

Patterned Wilton carpets are woven on a loom with a special device (a Jacquard), which enables one coloured thread at a time to be drawn up as pile, while the remaining threads are hidden in the backing of the carpet. It is unusual for there to be more than five colours as if there were, there would be a great deal of wastage of pile yarns carried along the backing. This method of manufacture lends itself to short but economic runs enabling establishments to have their own exclusive designs. Two-toned Wilton carpets are very usual.

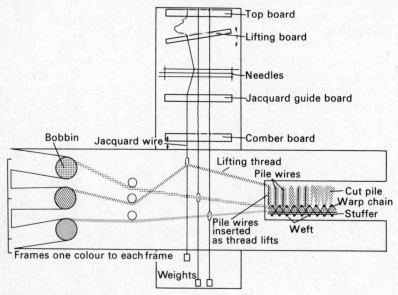

To show the working of a 3-frame Wilton loom

Owing to this method of construction, Wilton carpet has a firm, smooth back, with streaks of colour in it where the particular threads are not required as surface pile. The pile itself is close, confining spillages to the surface, varies in length even in the same carpet when a textured appearance results, and is sometimes made of curled yarns giving a short, twisted pile often referred to as a 'kinky' pile.

Plain Wilton carpets are made on a similar loom to the patterned, but without the Jacquard; extra jute threads, known as stuffers, fill the back of the carpet instead of the hidden coloured pile yarn. The backing still has the characteristic firmness.

Brussels carpets and cord carpets are variations of the Wilton weave in which the pile is uncut, i.e. looped. Brussels is an uncut patterned

Wilton and cord is an uncut plain Wilton. The latter was originally hair cord, i.e. made of a mixture of hair fibres from the horse, goat or cow but now quite frequently has rayon or cotton added, when it is not nearly so hardwearing but much cheaper. Looped or uncut pile carpets probably give 5–10% more wear than the same quality cut pile, but they have not the same softness or resilience as the cut pile carpets.

Axminster carpets in general are woven in such a way that the pile is almost entirely on the surface and the backing has a distinctive rib; no dead threads are carried in the backing and the pile is less close than in Wilton.

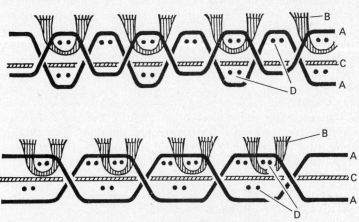

Gripper Axminster   Spool Axminster: (a) chain   (c) stuffer warp
                                            (b) pile   (d) double weft

Spool Axminster is probably the most popular type of carpet and can have an unlimited number of colours in the design. A characteristic of this type of carpet is that the pattern can be seen on the reverse side.

Gripper Axminster in appearance is similar to many spool Axmin-

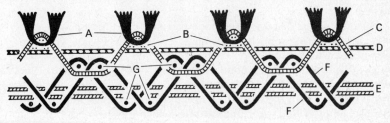

Chenille Axminster: (a) chenille fur   (d) float warp   (g) filler weft
                           (b) fur weft   (e) stuffer warp
                           (c) catcher warp   (f) chain

sters, but owing to its method of construction the number of colours is limited to twelve.

Chenille Axminster is quite unlike any carpet mentioned so far, but is still a woven carpet. In this case the pile is produced first as a long strip rather like a furry caterpillar (*chenille* is French for caterpillar), and during the weaving of the actual carpet, catcher threads attach these strips of pile to the backing. The catcher threads holding the pile can be seen quite distinctly in the finished carpet. The result is a soft, thick carpet with unlimited colours and design. It is, however, not produced in any quantity these days.

Oriental carpets are hand-woven carpets from the Middle and Far East. Machine-made copies of the genuine carpets are produced nowadays and these are not so hardwearing, and will naturally cost less. Genuine Oriental carpets are extremely hardwearing and the price of some increases with age, provided they are in good condition. There are carpets and rugs from Persia, India, China, etc., which are antiques and fetch colossal prices.

The pile of Oriental carpets may be of wool, silk or mixtures of these, and is made by the individual worker, knotting lengths of the yarn to the cotton warp threads of the hand loom, the type of knot differing slightly from place to place. There are, for example, Persian, Turkish and Gheordez knots.

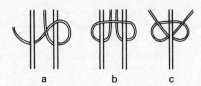

Typical hand-tied knots: (a) Persian (b) Turkish (c) Gheordez

Cotton threads form the weft as well as the warp in the backing and both vary in thickness from one carpet or rug to another. Oriental carpets are only made as carpet squares (over 213 cm x 121 cm) or rugs (under 213 cm x 121 cm), often having two fringed ends, and never as strip or body carpet.

Persian carpets or rugs were made originally as tapestry wall coverings, floor coverings on which people sat, or as prayer mats when there was a one way pattern. The patterns are generally all over, delicate, intricate and often of symbolic motifs, flowers and pine cones. Whole families, even several generations may contribute to the making of a Persian carpet with the result that irregularities in design and dye often occur. The dyes used are vegetable ones which are blended to produce a variety of beautiful subtle colours.

Indian carpets were generally made from coarser, longer pile than were other Oriental ones and less patterned than the Persian ones. There are of course many modern Indian ones on the market and some of these are of poor quality, tend to flatten and moult, but when they are of good quality they wear extremely well.

Chinese carpets have a close, silky pile with a well-defined pattern (not usually all over) often hand carved from the pile.

While Oriental carpets are not in normal use in establishments due to their cost, some may be found in the foyer or lounge of a luxury hotel or club, or in the manager's office. Repairs to these carpets can only be carried out by experts at great expense as the materials, colours and patterns all require skilled attention.

Modern Oriental carpets may be in use in some hotels.

Tufted carpets are made by a modern method of manufacture first introduced about 1946, in an attempt to produce a cheaper form of floor covering. The tufts or pile were originally of viscose rayon, but owing to its tendency to soil and flatten, this did not prove very satisfactory and blends of other man-made fibres and wool were used. Now, in addition to these blends there are tufted carpets of 100 per cent. synthetic fibre or 100 per cent. wool and consequently there is a very wide price range.

The pile is inserted into the backing by a long row of needles and may be cut or uncut. It is held in place by latex or PVC compounds. These enable tufted carpets to be cut to any shape without fraying, and pieces to be joined easily with adhesive tape. Stretching and buckling of the carpets were problems at first, but these have been largely overcome by a backing of hessian put on top of the adhesive. Designs are still limited although there has been notable advance in the last few years.

Adhesively bonded carpets and cloths are still newer than tufted carpets. In these the fibres are very dense and may form a conventional pile which is held in a PVC backing, or may be laid horizontally, resin bonded to a tough fibre base presenting a flat surface resembling needleloom felt (adhesively bonded cloths). The pile of the adhesively bonded carpets and cloths is normally of nylon or polypropylene but there is at least one type containing animal hair and this has to be sprayed with water occasionally to maintain the moisture content of the hair.

Adhesively bonded carpets have an appearance similar to a cut, close pile woven carpet, are extremely hardwearing and may be used in a variety of places. The bonded cloths of needleloom construction have not as good an appearance although they too are extremely hardwearing and may be considered as bridging the gap between the semi-hard floorings and the traditional type of carpet. Some of the adhesively bonded carpets and cloths may be laid as loose carpet tiles (approximately 45 cm) when the tiles may be moved periodically to even the wear.

Carpets and carpeting are made in varying widths depending on the weave and type of carpet. Broadloom carpets are woven on extra wide looms, and are normally between 2 m and 5 m wide but it is possible to get one variety as much as 10 m wide. Body or strip carpet is usually 68 cm or 90 cm wide, and is one which has no border so that the pattern matches when it is joined for fitted carpets (also called close fitted or wall to wall carpeting), i.e. where the floor is completely covered with carpet. The pile of a carpet lies slightly in one direction, so care must be taken when joining the carpet that the pile all lies in the same direction. If not, it is possible to get slight variations in shade.

A carpet square is a loose carpet with all edges neatened; it is not necessarily a square, but should strictly be over 210 cm x 120 cm. It does not fit the floor exactly and can be turned round to even the wear. A rug or mat is normally oblong, less than 210 cm x 120 cm, has all edges neatened and is often used in front of a fireplace or beside a bed.

Stair carpet often has a border and may be 45 cm, 56 cm, 68 cm or 90 cm wide, while broadloom carpeting can be used on a very wide staircase. These variations enable the same design to be used along corridors of different widths from the stairs. In the case of stair carpet, the pile should always run down the stairs (one sweeps with the pile, i.e. down the stairs), and an extra length should be bought to enable 'jogging', or moving of the carpet, to even the wear.

Carpets may be plain or patterned. A plain carpet makes a room look larger, and enables patterned materials to be used for other furnishings to better effect but it shows dirt, stains and crush marks (i.e. shading due to the bending of the pile) much more readily than a patterned one. When patterned, the design should be of a size which will not make the room appear small, and an all over design is probably the most serviceable as dirt, stains and crush marks will not show so easily. Carpets can be woven to any particular design or colour provided a sufficient length is being bought. Some carpet colours fade more readily than others but with improved dyes fading is not the problem it was.

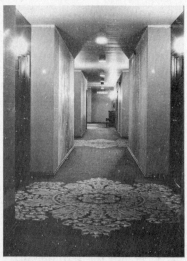

An example of the use of plain and patterned carpet

There is a tremendous price range in all types of carpets, and the more highly priced ones will obviously be chosen where there is much wear and tear unless it is a place where a constant change of décor is required. A good carpet should have a firm backing and pile anchorage, as well as a close resilient pile and a good quality carpet may have 20 tufts per cm². The choice of the grade of the carpet will be determined by the amount of wear and tear a given area will receive coupled with the life expectancy. The function of the area will therefore not only determine the desirability of using a certain texture or design but the weight or grade of the carpet as well.

For contract work three grades of carpet are suggested and the minimum pile weights generally recommended for hotel usage are as follows:

light contract, e.g. bedrooms	750–900 g
medium contract, e.g. lounges	1200–1350 g
heavy contract, e.g. entrances and student common rooms	1800–1950 g

It is wise before buying to have tests carried out for abrasion dynamic loading, compression recovery and to ascertain the analysis of the pile construction.

To obtain maximum wear from a carpet it must be well laid and this is a job for the expert. The subfloor should be smooth and dry, with no wide cracks in it or any protruding nails. A carpet may be stuck to the floor when it has been suggested that the carpet may last longer, but it means the carpet cannot be taken up and the good parts used elsewhere. When not stuck down a carpet underlay made of felt, rubber or synthetic foam is essential; it eliminates any slight unevenness in the floor, retards crushing and creeping, provides an extra layer of heat and sound insulation and makes the carpet feel soft and luxurious. By giving resilience it takes the strain of feet and lengthens the life of the carpet, but because of its great resilience it is wise to avoid rubber underlays (especially foam rubber) under a seamed carpet. Felts of natural fibres tend to pack down and lose their resilience in time and a felt and latex underlay combines many advantages of both rubber and felt. There are felts of 100 per cent. courtelle with good durability and resilience. The underlay should be the same size as the carpet and in the case of stairs if it is not continuous, the underlay should be in the form of pads which go right over the edge or nosing of the stair. When the underlay has a canvas backing or one smooth surface this is laid uppermost.

Stair and fitted carpets need fixing in some way, whereas a carpet square is generally laid loose on the floor. Stair carpets must be held

taut, and for a wide staircase rods
are better than clips and may be
used in conjunction with tackless
grippers. Carpet squares and rugs
can be backed with thin foam
rubber or rubberized net to
prevent them slipping.

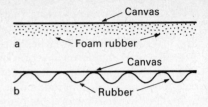

Suitable methods for fixing carpets

1   Tackless gripper—steel pins protrude from plywood strips fixed to
the floor or stairs, and hold the carpet in place. The edge of the carpet
is sometimes covered with another piece of wood.

2   Turn and tack—the edge of the carpet is turned under and tacks
put through the double surface but the carpet edge is inclined to ruckle
and lifting is difficult.

3   Sunken—the carpet is laid in a sunken area, the edges of which are
covered with brass or wood as for sunken front door mats.

4   Pin and socket
5   Ring and peg
6   Press studs
7   Touch and close fastener

These methods are especially suitable where a carpet needs lifting
frequently, e.g. banqueting rooms
cleared for dancing.

Where part of a carpet sometimes needs lifting a heavy duty zip
fastener or lacing can be used to fix it to the remaining carpet.

Druggets are used to protect carpets against dirt and excessive wear
in particular places at certain times, e.g. wet weather, redecoration, etc.
They are lengths of canvas laid as a covering over the carpet, so that
they take the dirt and wear instead of the carpet. Strips of canvas,
rubber or brass placed over the edge or nosing of the stair give protection to stair carpets at the place of greatest wear.

Other ways of preventing excessive wear in particular areas are by
the use of mats and by avoiding traffic lanes. The latter may be done
by turning the carpet (this may extend its life by as much as 5%), by
jogging the stair carpet or by having a flexible furniture arrangement.

Advantages of carpets

1   Carpets add to the decorative appearance of the room.
2   They can give a luxurious appearance and feel.
3   They are warm and may keep out draughts.
4   They are quiet and afford sound insulation.
5   They are non-slip.
6   Carpet squares and rugs break up a floor surface and can be
turned around.
7   Fitted carpets make a room look larger, and there is only one floor
surface to clean.

8   Patterned carpets do not show stains as much as plain ones.

Disadvantages
1   The surface holds dirt, so careful cleaning is necessary.
2   They are cut by grit and sharp castors and are burned or melted by cigarette ends.
3   They may be attacked by moth if of wool.
4   Shading can occur.
5   Fitted carpets show definite areas of wear.
6   Plain carpets show stains readily and stains can be difficult to remove *in situ*.
7   A large pattern for a fitted carpet is extravagant because of the need to match the pattern.
8   Initial cost of good carpet is high.

Grit is the worst enemy of carpets for it works its way into the base of the pile and appearances are deceptive. In some areas the grit may be removed by light cleaning when the vacuum cleaner is passed over the surface 2 or 3 times, or thorough vacuum cleaning may be required when up to 7 strokes are passed over the area; a carpet sweeper removes superficial crumbs and dust only. Damage by moth and carpet beetles may be the result of insufficient cleaning.

Periodic cleaning involves a room being out of use and obviously in most places this time is required to be as short as possible. Periodic cleaning is done *off site* or *in situ*. When done *off site* there is the expense of taking up and relaying, and the danger of shrinkage, but it is a more thorough clean. When done *in situ* the cleaning of a large carpet involves skilled labour and noisy machinery but it may be done by contractors many of whom offer a round-the-clock service.

In wet cleaning or shampooing, a detergent which dries to a non-sticky powder is advisable; it, with the held dirt, can then be picked up with a vacuum cleaner, the pile raised and the carpet left to dry. If the shampoo does not dry to a powder a sticky residue is left on the pile (particularly of man-made fibres) and this residue is difficult to remove and readily attracts soiling. In wet cleaning it is essential that the backing of the carpet does not become too wet so excess water should be avoided. Shampooing carpets will not kill all the micro-organisms which may be spread by humans and pets to the carpets, and in such areas as schools and especially hospitals frequent disinfecting of carpets is necessary to avoid the spreading of micro-organisms. Until recently, disinfectants available have led to changes in colour and the faster accumulation of dirt, but now one based on benzyl-hemiformal has been found which even after prolonged use does not cause fading or dirt accumulation.

The carpet may be treated during manufacture or during shampooing or the spread of micro-organisms can be prevented almost entirely by daily spray-vacuum cleaning when by means of a suitable spraying device attached to the vacuum cleaner the disinfecting fluid is sprayed into the pile of the carpet.

In dry cleaning an inert powdered material saturated with either a grease solvent or a detergent is spread over the surface of the carpet and then picked up with a vacuum cleaner. The surface of the carpet is brightened but the cleaning is not as thorough as when the carpet is wet cleaned; there is, however, less likelihood of shrinkage and the room is available for use more quickly.

Synthetic fibres tend to build up static electricity (although epitropic fibres are now being produced) so anti-static finishes may be given to the surface or anti-static fibres of stainless steel or copper may be introduced into the fibre or pile of a carpet to reduce the risk of electric shocks. Anti-static finishes may include anti-soiling properties.

Carpets may also be given water and stain resistant finishes. These are surface treatments which have little effect on the texture or the appearance of the carpets, but provide a barrier between the fibre and the spillage. Similar treatments may be given to upholstery coverings.

Care and cleaning

1 Have a smooth, even subfloor.
2 Use a good underlay.
3 Do not use a rubber underlay for a seamed carpet.
4 Vacuum clean frequently.
5 Brush or use vacuum cleaner attachments on the edges of the carpet at frequent intervals.
6 Avoid vacuum cleaning woollen carpets when very new to allow loose fibres to felt (bed down).
7 Remove stains as soon as possible (for more unusual stains, see Chapter 4).
8 Take care of rubber backing when using dry cleaning fluid.
9 Shampoo when necessary.
10 Protect damp carpet from castors and metal legs of furniture.
11 Protect carpet with drugget or hearth cloth when necessary.
12 Use nosing on stairs.
13 Attend to any shifting of the carpet.
14 Attend to showing underlay.
15 Prevent rugs from creeping by use of foam rubber or rubberised net.
16 Secure edges of carpets at doorways and staircases.
17 Protect against damage by moth if not already mothproofed.
18 Attend to wear from sharp castors.
19 Repair frayed edges and worn parts.
20 Cut off loose ends, particularly looped, never pull pile.
21 Jog stair carpet and move carpet squares regularly.

Matting

Matting can be made from a variety of materials and the appearance and wearing quality depends on the materials from which it is manufactured. Coconut fibre, sisal, wood fibre, jute and rush are woven or plaited to form matting. In addition strips of plastic are being used. In all cases, because of the loose weave, dirt filters through the matting to the floor below, thus necessitating the frequent lifting of the mats, so that the dirt may be removed.

Front door mats made from jute and coconut fibres do much to save the foyer or entrance hall from dirt. They should have a firm edge as this is the place which wears, and once worn the pile falls out.

Advantages
Front door mats save the floor from much dirt.

Disadvantages
1 Dirt filters through.
2 If large they are heavy to move.
3 Good quality is expensive.

Care and cleaning
1 Attend to worn or frayed edges.
2 Front doormat—lift, turn upside down and tread on it to force dirt out. Remove dust from well before relaying.

Plastic matting—sweep or vacuum clean and occasionally lift and sweep under. Wash when necessary.

Other matting—sweep with a hard broom or vacuum clean and occasionally lift and sweep under. Scrub when necessary.

9

Wall Coverings

The function of a wall covering may be purely decorative when the ability to bring colour, pattern, texture, light or shade to the room may be of the greatest importance; on the other hand the covering may be required to give an easily cleaned and hygienic surface. From the great variety of available wall coverings, the choice is very wide but at all times the style should suit the purpose, the furnishings and the architectural aspects of the room.

Another point for consideration is whether the wall covering is required to last a long time and thus may have more money spent on it or whether the general décor will be changed more frequently and so a less expensive covering should be chosen. In addition, the wall covering must comply with the fire regulations.

In most cases the flooring would be more expensive and outlast the wall covering so the latter should take second place. There is also often a larger expanse of wall noticeable and less broken surface than on the floor, so wall coverings should blend with, rather than dominate, the general scheme. The need for warmer and more intimate interiors has led to the increasing use of textured wall coverings.

It is possible to introduce more than one type of wall covering into a room. In this way impact colours, designs or materials can be used for focal points to add interest (see Chapter 12), or areas where there is likely to be the greatest wear and tear can have the most durable surface, and choice will then be made on account of resistance to abrasion, tearing, etc., as well as frequent cleaning.

Wall coverings inevitably become very rubbed and scratched by the movement of chairs, the carrying of luggage, the banging of trolleys and the rubbing caused by people as they pass. It is possible to guard against the marking of the wall in various ways, for example:

1 By using a stronger and more easily cleaned material for the lower part of the wall, possibly up to 150 cm, when this is called a dado.
2 By fixing narrow strips of wood to the floor or even to the wall, in such a way that chairs are not pushed right against the wall.
3 By using glass, perspex or melamine plastics as a protective mate-

rial in vulnerable places, such as around light switches or walls against which people lean or which trolleys damage.

4   By fixing doorstops.

Wall coverings should be used on suitably prepared walls.

Preparation of the walls often involves quite a lot of work and this adds considerably to the labour costs, as in some cases the preparation entails more labour than the actual application of the new covering. The curing of the cause of any dampness, the filling of cracks and holes, the removal of dirt and the build up of old paint and old papers are but a few of the jobs involved in preparation.

Paints

Paint is used extensively as a wall finish when it is used primarily for decoration, but it is also used to preserve and protect structural surfaces, especially those of wood and metal; it can be used for identification of pipes, for the emphasis of hazards and danger points, and for hygiene, as paint facilitates the cleaning of surfaces.

As a wall covering paint offers a wide choice of types, colours and degrees of gloss and even design if murals are painted on to the walls. Whatever covering is chosen for the walls, gloss paint is normally used as a protective coating for window frames and sills, doors and skirting boards and in many instances it gives a contrast in colour and texture to the main wall finish so contributing to the décor of the room.

It is hoped that maintenance painting will last several years and the cost should be calculated per year and not per job. Using cheaper or more expensive paint does not affect the total cost of the job significantly as labour costs will account for the greater part of the total cost (i.e. labour and material costs), but the choice may have a great effect on the durability of the painted surface and labour costs may be saved over the years. Thus a more expensive paint may last 4 years instead of 3 without increasing the cost per job greatly and the cost per year may be decreased, e.g. a £900–job lasting 3 years costs £300 per year; if £1,000 is spent and the job lasts 4 years, cost per year is £250 only.

Paint used for a wall finish is normally required for decoration rather than protection, but there is a need for washability, as all paints (except multicolour paints) tend to attract dust. (Stretch level dusting can in time become very noticeable and unless walls are washed from bottom to top, drip marks result on the dry surface and these are difficult to remove later.)

Paint is relatively cheap, easily applied and cleaned; it can give textural and multicoloured effects but it shows soiling (especially matt paints) and wall imperfections (especially gloss paints) more readily than other wall coverings. Although there are quick drying and low smelling paints, drying time and the lingering odour must be remembered when considering the time a room has to be 'off' for redecoration.

The main types of paints used as wall finishes are:

Water paints and distempers

As the name implies these are water thinned and due to their poor durability have been superseded by emulsion paints.

Emulsion paints

These are also water thinned but are based on dispersions of synthetic resins (e.g. polyvinyl acetate) which dry to tough, washable and wear resistant films. Emulsion paints are available in a wide range of colours and various degrees of sheen from matt to semi-gloss. Vinyl gloss paint is now available. Being alkali-resistant, they are suitable for use on new, possibly damp plaster, etc. They are quick drying and low in odour, and so are very suitable for redecoration of rooms which cannot remain long out of use.

Alkyd paints

These are based on synthetic (alkyd) resins combined with a vegetable oil, such as linseed oil. In finishing paints, alkyd paints have almost completely replaced the older types based on natural resins, although the latter are still used in primers and undercoating paints. Alkyd paints are generally easier to apply, and have better durability and wearing properties than the older types. The use of modern pigments ensures good opacity, and excellent light fastness in a wide range of colours. Polyurethane is sometimes included to give a more scratch resistant surface.

Alkyd paints are available as gloss, eggshell and flat finishes. Some types are supplied as thixotropic or 'jelly' paints which are claimed not to splash, drip or run, and to permit heavy application for maximum obliteration.

Clear polyurethane paints are like a varnish, but it is only possible to get a matt finish on wood.

Multi-colour paints

These are usually dispersions of cellulose colours in water. Each colour is present in separate 'blobs' or 'spots', the resulting effect being dependent on the number of different colours, the degree of contrast between them, and the size and distribution of the 'spots'. Usually this type of paint must be spray-applied. It is extremely hardwearing and the multi-colour effect helps to mask surface irregularities and imperfections. Corridors, entrance halls, hospital wards, cloakrooms and toilets are ideal places in which to use this type of finish.

Texture or 'plastic' paints

These are usually plaster-based and are intended to give a textured or relief effect on the surface. The texture is obtained by working over the material, after application and while it is still wet, using combs, palette knives, strippers, etc., and much depends on the skill and taste of the operative. Some types are self-coloured, others may require painting when they are dry.

A modern type of texture material is based on a heavy bodied synthetic resin emulsion, and may be applied by spray, direct to concrete and similar surfaces thus eliminating the need for plastering. Such coatings are very tough and hard wearing, and their principal usage is similar to that of the multi-colour finishes.

There are paints with special properties, e.g. insecticidal, fire retardant, etc., and these may be advantageously used in certain places.

Care and cleaning of painted surfaces

1 Remove light dust with a duster, wall broom or vacuum cleaner attachments.

2 Wash when necessary, with warm water and suitable detergent to remove heavily ingrained or tenacious dust and dirt. This is important on low sheen surfaces as dry cleaning tends to force dust into the surface. Distempers and water paints will not withstand much soaking or scrubbing, but the 'washable' types can usually be sponged down lightly.

3 When washing, start from the bottom and work upwards, using a sponge or worn distemper brush. Change the solution frequently. Rinse from the top downwards, using frequent changes of water. Sponge dry. Washing down is normally a maintenance job.

4 Low sheen finishes, especially emulsion paints, may tend to 'polish up' if isolated areas of bad soiling are rubbed vigorously with a damp cloth. Clean such areas by very lightly scrubbing with a damp nail brush and a little fine scouring powder, when the dirt should be removed without damage or 'polishing'.

5 Never apply wax polishes or oil to gloss painted surfaces to 'revive' them. The residues may cause subsequent paint coatings to peel, or fail to dry.

6 Do not use harsh abrasives, strong solvents or strong soda solutions to clean paintwork, or the film may be damaged or softened.

Wallpaper

Most wallpapers in this country are made in rolls of 10 m x 53 cm, but many foreign ones vary in length and width. The price varies enormously, depending on the quality of the design and the materials used.

Wallpaper may be smooth or have a textured effect introduced. This may be done by the superimposing or interlayering of other substances to give a rough surface, or by clever designing when apparent depth (three-dimensional effect) may result. A smooth finish to the paper is more resistant to dust than when the surface is rough but marks generally show more. The pattern may be of many kinds: floral, geometric, abstract, striped, etc., of two or more colours, and in many cases is an all over design. The choice should depend on the aspect, height, size and use of the room. Vertical, horizontal, receding and advancing designs and colours can all affect the apparent architectural features of the room. Large patterned papers tend to overpower and make a small room appear smaller; they also cut to waste owing to the need for matching the pattern. Most wallpapers have a warmer appearance than paint and offer some sound insulation. Patterned and textured wallpapers cover up blemishes better, but where the walls are not 'true' a pattern causes problems and in any position a wrong choice of pattern can be very irritating. (Repainting is easier and less expensive than repapering.)

Pattern is added to paper by:

1   Wood block or hand printing—the paper is stamped with prepared blocks dipped in dye. This paper is expensive.

2   Screen printing—prepared silk screens are used as stencils.

3   Roller printing or intaglio—the paper is printed by engraved rollers which may give an embossed effect.

4   Photogravure—photographic reproductions of wood grain and similar designs.

New walls are not normally papered at first as it is wiser to allow them to dry out completely; however, paper gives a warmer appearance than paint and can hide many defects in the wall. In order to withstand steamy atmospheres and be spongeable, suitable papers may be treated during manufacture or after application to the wall, thus making wallpaper suitable for almost any type of room except perhaps large kitchens, laundries and hospital wards.

Wallpapers may become soiled, scratched and torn with abrasion more easily than many other wall coverings. It is possible to stick back torn and peeling pieces, and as mentioned earlier, some protection may be given to vulnerable places. In addition to the conventional wallpapers there are now available many paper-backed materials, e.g. fabrics, wood veneers and plastics, etc., which are being hung in a similar way to the conventional papers. Some of these newer coverings are extremely resistant to scratching, tearing and cleaning, and may be considered as being too durable and too expensive for areas where the décor is likely to be changed frequently.

Some types of wallpaper

1 Ordinary surface printed papers.

2 Spongeable papers are those specially treated during manufacture to withstand water.

3 Anaglypta is an embossed or raised pattern paper. It is hollow backed and often used as a dado or as ceiling paper.

4 Oatmeal papers are those where texture is produced by the inter-layering of wood dust, chopped straw or similar material during manufacture.

5 Flock papers are papers treated with adhesive to which silk, wool, cotton or man-made fibres (the flocking) stick to give a raised pile.

6 Wood grain papers are photographic reproductions of various wood grains and waxed during manufacture.

7 Metallic papers are those printed with gold and other metallic powders.

8 Silk papers are silk or silk-like fabrics backed with paper.

9 Grass papers are woven grasses or similar materials mounted on paper.

10 Wood veneer papers are thin veneers of wood mounted on paper.

11 Cork papers are thin veneers of cork mounted on paper.

12 Plastic surfaced papers (see plastic wall coverings).

Lincrusta is a paper-backed textured composition, frequently simulating wood panelling.

Cleaning of wallpapers

1 Remove surface dust with a wall broom or vacuum cleaner attachments (low suction for flock papers).

2 Remove marks by rubbing with a soft india rubber or a piece of soft bread. If the paper is spongeable, wipe with a damp cloth or sponge.

3 Attempt to remove grease with a proprietary grease absorber but it may prove difficult to do so satisfactorily.

Other Wall Coverings

Plastic wall coverings

Many types of plastic wall coverings are available now and they are becoming increasingly popular; some are more decorative than others and some afford sound insulation, but all, owing to their abrasion resistance, are more hardwearing and easily cleaned than most other wall coverings. They are obtainable in a variety of sizes with a great price range and many require special adhesives. As they are non-porous there is a greater tendency for the growth of moulds so the adhesive should contain fungicides, or a fungicidal wash used on the wall prior to hanging the plastic wall covering.

Vinyl is the most usual plastic and normally coats paper or woven fabric. It may be used to resemble silk, tweed or other fabrics as well as wood, stone or brick.

Some types of plastic wall coverings

1 Plastic (PVC) surfaced papers or fabrics, e.g. Vymura, Baladore, Fablon, etc.
2 Vinyl flock papers.
3 Plastic cloths.
4 Padded PVC material used as panelling, e.g. Panaquil.
5 Laminated plastic produced as surface boards or as a veneer which requires sticking to plywood. Melamine is the resin frequently used during the manufacture of these plastic laminates which may simulate wood panelling or fabrics, e.g. Formica, Warerite, etc.
6 Plastic wall tiles imitate ceramic tiles.
7 Expanded polystyrene in sheet or tile form used on walls and ceilings to give heat and sound insulation, and to help eliminate condensation. It can be painted with emulsion paint or covered with paper. It is dissolved by spirit based paints and thus before the use of oil paint it should be lined with paper and given a coat of emulsion paint to act as a buffer.

Cleaning of plastic wall coverings
1 Remove surface dust with duster, wall broom or vacuum cleaner attachments.
2 Wash, when necessary, with warm water and synthetic detergent. A soft brush may be used on these surfaces.

Fabric wall coverings

It is possible to cover a wall with any fabric and its durability will depend on the fibre and weave used in its manufacture. The fabrics may be hung loosely or they may be attached to a frame which is secured to the wall, while some fabrics may be paper-backed or specially prepared so that they can be actually stuck to the wall. Fabrics hung in loose folds are useful when dealing with difficult wall surfaces and covering ugly features. Fabrics may bring warmth and better acoustic properties to an area while their sound-deadening properties help against noise in adjoining rooms. Those chosen should not be liable to sag, buckle or stretch when hung permanently on the wall or collect excessive dust or dirt. Dust and the smell of smoke tend to cling to fabrics with a pile or rough surface more than to smooth fabrics.

Wild silk and other beautiful fabrics may be padded for heat and sound insulation, and for effect they may be stretched taut, gathered or pleated into a frame. Silks and tapestries are expensive wall coverings and thus are more usually found in luxury establishments while hessian, linen and some acetate/viscose fabrics are cheaper and used more extensively.

The word 'tapestry' is frequently misused and applied to cross stitch (gros point) work on chair seats and stools, whereas true tapestry is a woven fabric and when used as a wall covering generally depicts a scene and hangs loosely on the wall, e.g. the tapestry in Coventry Cathedral. It should be remembered that wool materials may be attacked by moth and adequate precautions taken.

Cleaning of fabric wall coverings
1   Remove surface dust by brushing or vacuum cleaner attachments.
2   For the more beautiful hangings, when necessary dismantle and send to a firm of dry cleaners who specialise in this type of work.
3   Where hessian is stuck to the wall, scrub very lightly using warm water and synthetic detergent where necessary.

Wood panelling

Woods used for panelling are usually hard, well seasoned and of a decorative appearance, and they may cover the wall completely or form a dado. Wood panelling may be solid or veneered; it lasts for years with little maintenance providing precautions are taken in respect of dry rot and wood worm, but the initial cost is rather high. Wood veneers may be stuck to paper when they give a similar effect to the solid wood at much less cost and veneered plywood panelling is also available. Wood panelling may be used in such places as entrance halls and staircases, assembly halls, boardrooms and restaurants.

Cleaning of wood panelling
1   Dust and polish if necessary.
2   Where the panelling has become dirty or greasy wipe over with white spirit or vinegar and water and repolish.

Glass wall coverings

Glass can be used in the form of decorative tiles sometimes in the form of mosaics, and these should not be confused with glass bricks which allow the passage of light and form the wall itself. Coloured opaque glass sheets or tiles are often used as a wall covering in hotel bathrooms.

Glass as a wall covering is frequently used in the form of mirrors which are plate glass backed with a coating of coloured metallic paint, usually silver, and this reflects the light and can alter the apparent size of the room or passage. Mirrors may be above the dado or may cover the whole wall; they may be framed or unframed or in the form of tiles when they are sometimes 'antique' mirror giving a duller surface and there is less reflection. Mirrors are used in a great variety of places, e.g. foyers, restaurants, ballrooms and bathrooms.

There is available now a glass-less mirror (Mirralite) which has the advantage of not misting up or shattering and is about 1/5 of the weight of conventional mirror. It consists of a polyester film vacuum coated with aluminium and mounted on a flat frame.

Cleaning of glass
1 Dust or wipe with a damp chamois leather or scrim. Proprietary cleansers or methylated spirit may be used.
2 Care should be taken when cleaning mirrors that the backs do not become damp.

Metal wall coverings

Metals may be used for their decorative and their hygienic qualities.

Metals such as copper and anodised aluminium are decorative and may be used for effect in such areas as bars where the metal in combination with rows of bottles and interesting lighting can be most impressive. Other metals, usually stainless steel in the form of tiles, may be used in kitchens where they present a durable, easily cleaned hygienic surface in areas where splashing is likely.

Metal skirting boards provide coved edges between wall and floor surfaces. Metal foil can be elegant if used sparingly as a wall covering; it is available in a variety of colours.

Cleaning of metal wall coverings
1 Dust or wipe with a damp cloth.
2 Polish is not necessary on these metals as they either do not tarnish or have been treated against it.

Leather (hide) wall coverings

Leather wall coverings are extremely expensive and very decorative. They may be padded and studded with brass studs and would not be used to cover a complete wall surface. They may be found in luxury establishments in parts of the restaurants or bars, but are too expensive to be found in most places and in these, the effects of leather are simulated by plastics.

Cleaning of leather wall coverings
1 Remove surface dust by dusting, or vacuum cleaner attachments especially for the studded variety.
2 Apply cream polish sparingly and rub up very well.

Many flooring materials can be used as wall coverings. They contribute different colours, patterns and textures depending on the particular material. They are hardwearing, abrasion resistant and initially rather expensive. Some of them are particularly hygienic, easily cleaned surfaces and found in such places as kitchens, cloakrooms and bathrooms.

Amongst the floorings used as wall coverings there are:

marble	linoleum
terrazzo	cork
ceramic tiles	carpet

(For further details regarding cleaning see Chapter 7.)

Ceilings

Colour, pattern and texture can be introduced into ceilings, and they, as walls, have the ability to affect the space, light, heat and acoustic properties as well as the appearance of the room. It stands to reason that the manner in which the ceiling is treated should be in harmony with the general décor.

The original ceiling of a room is generally plastered and on to this almost any material may be put.

The ceiling may be papered, painted, decorated with wood in the form of beams or close slats, covered with tiles—acoustic, insulating or glass, including mirror, and in some special areas highly decorative mosaics are found as are other materials, e.g. nails used for decoration.

Panels can interrelate with the main material or perforated panels may allow the inset of other materials. In the former case use can be made of louvred woods, bamboo canes and metal grilles for example and in the latter grass cloths and other papers and fabrics may be used.

In some rooms suspended ceilings are useful and it is possible to introduce two-level ceilings in one room. Suspended ceilings are normally sheets of material supported on some form of framework and they offer a good opportunity for decorative effects although their purpose may be to hide ugly details, e.g. lighting and ventilating fittings, pipes, etc. They may give better proportions in the room or emphasise a particular area, provide better acoustic effect, form an interesting lighting effect, as well as create a purely decorative effect. The design should be for ease of cleaning and the maintenance of light fittings.

Cleaning of ceilings
1   Remove dust and cobwebs with a ceiling broom.
2   Where possible use vacuum extension for mouldings.

Beds and Bedding

When *guests* stay in an establishment they naturally are concerned with eating and sleeping, and the comfort of the beds is of great importance to them. The beds must not only be comfortable but must look inviting, and this will depend on the design, the materials from which they are made, and the neatly finished appearance of the beds in the room.

In the past beds have normally been 6 ft or 6 ft 3 in in length and 2 ft 6 in, 3 ft or 3 ft 3 in wide for a single bed and 4 ft 6 in or 5 ft wide for a double bed but with the tendency of the modern generation to be taller and the implementing of metrication, standards are likely to be:

100 x 200 cm (3 ft 3⅜ in x 6 ft 6¾ in)
85 x 190 cm (2 ft 9½ in x 6 ft 3 in)
150 x 200 cm (4 ft 11 in x 6 ft 6¾ in)
135 x 190 cm (4 ft 5 in x 6 ft 3 in)

and there are larger ones known as King size. As beds are individually made it is possible for establishments to get a quotation for sizes other than the standard ones.

A bed consists of a mattress supported by a base. The base may be of open coiled springs, wire mesh, laminated wood strips, or the coiled springs may be padded and covered to give an upholstered base. Ticking is the usual covering but the sides may be covered in PVC for easier cleaning. Added strength is sometimes given to the base by reinforcing the edge, while in other cases the edge is raised to enable the mattress to be dropped in. This type of base is often used for students' beds because not only does it prevent damage when the bed is sat on but it prevents the mattress from slipping off and therefore gives a tidier appearance; it does, however, make bedmaking more difficult.

When the base is not upholstered, there should be an underlay of strong material such as hessian or canvas to protect the mattress from abrasion. The base may be surrounded by a valance and an upholstered one, when not covered in PVC, by a base cover. The height of the bed will influence the ease with which an elderly *guest* can get in and out of it, the ease with which it can be made and lastly the appearance of the bed in the room. There are beds in some hospitals with a lifting

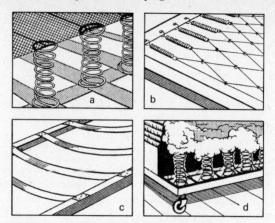

Bed bases: (a) open coiled springs (b) stretched springs
(c) laminated wood strips (d) upholstered

mechanism which enables the beds to be raised for making, clinical procedures, etc., and lowered to enable the patient to get in and out more easily.

It is usual for a bed to have a headboard, though this may be fixed to the wall and the bed pushed against it, as is the case with divans. The headboard must be sufficiently high (30–45 cm above the top of the mattress) to protect the wall from soiling when *guests* sit up in bed. In hospitals, bedsteads are usual and the metal headboard is normally adjustable to give a back rest for greater comfort. In other places headboards may be of different materials such as wood, metal or plastic and where necessary polished, painted or padded. They may be made in plain or fancy shapes and may incorporate a bedside table, light switches and even a telephone. There may or may not be a footboard but, in any case, foot- and headboards must be firm to prevent movement and squeaking. The feet of the bed should be such that they will neither scratch a polished surface, nor damage a carpet by cutting or badly flattening it, nor move too readily when the *guest* is in bed. Suitable castors should therefore be used, such as small wheels which may lock, steel skids, etc.

A divan is normally a low bed without a head- or footboard, may or may not be upholstered and can be used as a bed at night and converted into a settee by day and thus is used in studio rooms and study bedrooms when a drawer in the base can prove extremely useful.

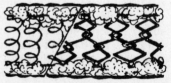

Section through upholstered mattress showing (a) coiled springs; (b) posture springing

Mattresses

Mattresses are nowadays basically interior sprung, latex or plastic foam. There were stuffed mattresses filled with hair, hair and wool or flock. Good hair is expensive; flock is cheap but becomes lumpy and all stuffed mattresses are absorbent and liable to attack by moth and other pests. They require frequent turning when in use and remaking every few years and thus these mattresses have in many places been replaced by the interior sprung, latex or plastic foam ones.

Interior sprung mattresses are made of a continuous wire construction (posture springing) or of coiled springs of tempered wire very firmly held in position, and there may be different grades of springs in different parts of the mattress, so giving more even support to the body when lying on them. The springs are well padded with layers of cotton waste, coiled hair, rubber or plastic foam, and the whole is then tightly covered with a strong ticking. Before the introduction of rubber or plastic foam into the padding, the cotton waste, wool and hair were held firmly in place by string pulled through at regular intervals and held by buttons, pieces of leather or tufts of wool on the top and bottom of the mattress. This tufting collects dust and can be uncomfortable to lie on and now buttonless mattresses, where there is a top layer of rubber or plastic foam immediately below the ticking, are available. Quilting is another means of anchoring the fillings.

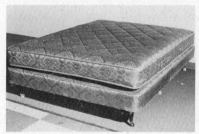 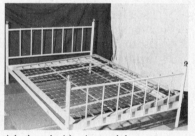

A divan with upholstered base and mattress   A bedstead with wire-mesh base

Interior sprung mattresses should have a reinforced edge for added strength. They vary in depth (12 cm–22 cm approx.), quality and price according to the number and gauge of springs, type of padding and quality of covering. To keep them in good condition they should be turned occasionally to even the wear. There are normally eyelet holes and handles on the sides of the mattress, the former to allow circulation of air and the latter to assist in turning. Interior sprung mattresses are heavy, absorbent and liable to attack by moth and other pests, but are comfortable and will last for many years.

Rubber mattresses are normally made from latex foam. The latex, which has previously been whisked with a chemical setting agent, is poured into heated moulds where it is shaped, set and vulcanised, without losing any of its tiny air cells. The mattress may be about 10 cm deep, and it normally has a right and wrong side due to the shape of the moulds and so should not be turned.

Deeper rubber mattresses have a specially developed foam base bonded on, but are still less deep and less heavy than interior sprung mattresses. As they are non-absorbent and return to their original shape after being lain on, they require no turning. They do not make dust or fluff, and are not liable to attack by moth and other pests.

Plastic mattresses are made from foam plastic, generally of the polyethylene type. Foam plastic mattresses are non-absorbent, make no dust or fluff, and are not liable to attack by moth and other pests.

There is a danger that when foam rubber and some foam plastic mattresses catch fire they produce fumes which are toxic, and although they may be treated this adds considerably to the price.

The British Standards Institute lays down minimum requirements for mattresses.

Care and cleaning of beds
1   Check for loose headboards.
2   Check divan legs screwed in tightly.
3   Check mattress does not sag and buttons or other tufting are not missing.
4   Check for soiling and tears in ticking.
5   Turn interior sprung mattresses occasionally, both sides and top to bottom to ensure even wear.
6   Use underlays on bases of open spring type.
7   Supply waterproof sheet for young children and other necessary occasions.
8   Fit base covers where upholstered bases not covered with PVC.
9   Dust or brush open wire springs occasionally.
10   Vacuum upholstered bases and mattresses.
11   Have valances and base covers laundered or dry cleaned when necessary.

Pillows

The most usual size for pillows is 48 cm x 73 cm and they consist of various fillings, covered with a strong closely woven material, ticking, which was formerly striped and is now more often white.

They may be filled with:

Down which comes from the breast of the duck, is expensive and very comfortable, and is liable to attack by moth.

Small feathers which are less expensive and less soft than down. They give a very satisfactory pillow but like down, are attacked by moth. There are down/feather combinations.

Rubber } The comments given for the mattresses also apply to
Plastic foam } pillows. However, many people find them too resilient for comfort.

Man-made fibres, e.g. terylene, which are bulked to give a soft handle, are expensive, moth proof and extremely comfortable.

Kapok, which comes from the cotton tree and not from the cotton plant, is soft at first but with use tends to become powdery and lose its softness and so is not a satisfactory filling; before the introduction of terylene filled rubber or plastic foam pillows kapok filled pillows were provided for guests with an allergy to feathers but are now seldom used. Kapok must not be confused with flock which owing to its lumpiness is not now used for pillows.

Bolsters

Bolsters are elongated pillows which stretch the width of the bed.

They form an underpillow, and as the head does not rest on them directly, they may be filled with a less resilient filling than pillows. They have gone out of fashion, and now a *guest* is normally given two pillows on the bed.

Care and cleaning of pillows
1 Shake feather pillows daily.
2 Repair splits or tears in the ticking immediately.
3 Protect with an underpillow slip.
4 Have dry cleaned or laundered if necessary, with the exception of rubber and plastic foam which may be wiped clean.

Blankets

People expect to be warm in bed, and it is usual to provide one under blanket (sometimes called bedpad) and two or three top blankets for each bed. The size of the blankets varies tremendously but they are generally a little shorter than sheets, e.g. 177 cm x 254 cm single, 228 cm x 254 cm double, as they do not require tucking in top and bottom. They are obtainable in the normal weave or in an open weave i.e. cellular.

White or pale coloured blankets are more often used in hotels thus enabling the guests to judge the standard of cleanliness when they are sleeping in strange beds. The top or bottom edges of a blanket may be stitched with a white or coloured wool (blanket stitched), or have a coloured binding to match. This binding may be of a man-made fibre and it gives a luxurious finish to the blanket. It is, however, expensive to replace when it frays.

Some reserve of blankets should be kept; these should be covered to keep them clean and if made of wool precautions taken against moth.

Blankets may be made of:

Wool. These are liable to attack by moth, are very warm and absorbent; they are expensive to launder and do not stand up to frequent laundering as they are liable to become harsh and felted so for hygienic reasons people sleep between sheets. Wool blankets get worn in time and the old ones are frequently used as underblankets; these are often folded and if not long enough to cover the whole length of the bed, they should reach from the pillow to the foot of the bed.

Synthetic fibres, e.g. acrilan, nylon, etc. These are very light and warm but rather expensive, and owing to their low moisture absorbency are very easily laundered without fear of felting. Acrilan blankets have been known to withstand 30 washings very satisfactorily and this could represent laundering twice a year for 15 years. Acrilan or nylon fibres are sometimes used in 'lace' blankets e.g. Moonweave, when the blankets are extremely light in weight.

Mixtures. Wool/cotton and wool/rayon and wool/nylon blankets are cheaper than wool, and more fluffy and attractive in appearance than cotton. As much care has to be taken of them in laundering as with wool blankets and in time the fluffiness of the wool wears but there is a reduction of felting and shrinkage.

Cotton. These are in a cellular form and are used in hospitals because of the frequent washing and boiling needed to prevent cross infection.

Underblankets are not normally provided on hospital beds and the plastic mattress covers often used, lead to a build-up of static electricity and shocks may be felt when the metal bedstead is touched at the same time.

In use, blankets become soiled, especially under blankets, and so will require to be laundered or dry cleaned. All blankets can be washed, but woollen ones are liable to felt and shrink and so for preference should be dry cleaned, however this is too expensive for the majority of establishments. In order that blankets are maintained in a 'spotless' condition, a blanket book is sometimes kept to record their cleaning, as a blanket may have to go to be cleaned out of turn because of a spill or other accident.

Electric blankets (see p. 42) are provided in some hotels.

Care and cleaning of blankets
1. Take precautions against moth in storing woollen blankets.
2. Repair frayed ends.

3. Check for stains and dirty marks.
4. Shake occasionally.
5. Have laundered or dry cleaned at regular intervals, or when necessary.

Eiderdowns and Quilts

Eiderdowns are filled with down which, strictly speaking, should be from the eider duck but owing to the expense of down, they are often filled with curled feathers, man-made fibres or other materials, and should then be spoken of as quilts, and the term 'quilt' is now used to cover all types.

Quilts provide a warm, light bed covering but are too expensive, initially and in upkeep, for many establishments. In hotels with central heating it may be considered unnecessary to provide them in addition to blankets. They may be covered with fabrics which are slippery (these in the main are made from man-made fibres) and the quilts then tend to slip off the bed; in order to counteract this, the underside may be made from a less slippery material, e.g. cotton sateen or brushed nylon. Another method to secure them on the bed, is to sew flaps of material on to either side of the quilt and to tuck these in, under the mattress. Quilts are generally placed under the bedspread and under the fold of the top sheet to keep them as clean as possible and to avoid tea and coffee stains which are difficult to remove from coloured fabrics. The sizes are approximately 84 cm x 127 cm and 144 cm x 127 cm.

Continental quilts filled with down or synthetic fibres are being used in some hotels. They may be used with a bottom sheet only when a clean cover for the quilt has to be provided for each new guest. The covers are more expensive to have laundered than a top sheet and maids find little time saved when covers have to be changed frequently (possibly daily). To overcome these problems a top sheet is provided with the quilt in some hotels.

Care and cleaning of quilts
1 Take precautions against moth in the storing of feather filled quilts.
2 Attend to repairs.
3 Check for stains and dirty marks.
4 Have feather filled quilts dry cleaned and others laundered.

Bedspreads

Bedspreads are used to cover the bed during the day, and may be removed at night, folded and put away. The colour and pattern must suit the décor of the room, matching, contrasting or picking up a colour

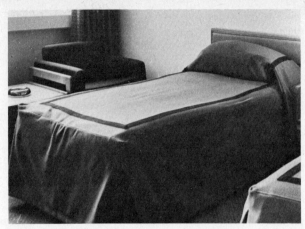

Fitted bedspread brought forward over the pillows

from the curtains or carpet. The bedspread is frequently sat on, has parcels put on it and may be folded nightly, so the material from which it is made should not crease or snag, and should stand up to frequent laundering or dry cleaning. Of the many materials suitable, some of the more commonly used are candlewick, taffeta, chintz, rayon and cotton satin and tapestry (see Chapter 5) and in hospitals heavy cotton fabrics.

Bedspreads may be of the fitted or throw-over type; the latter reaches almost to the ground and in order that the corners do not hang too low at the foot of the bed they may be rounded.

The throw-over bedspread can be held in place under the pillow, and then carried over it to the back of the bed. Alternatively the pillow may be placed on top of the bedspread to which a reverse piece of material, about 114 cm in length has been attached, and this is brought forward and tucked under the pillow.

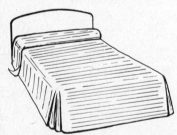
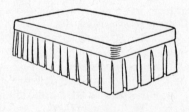

A throw-over type of bedspread with the corners 'rounded'   Fitted bedspread on divan without pillows

In the case of fitted bedspreads the top is of the exact size of the bed plus bedding, and the sides may be quite straight, pleated or frilled to within an inch of the floor. The top of the bedspread can be finished as for the top of the throw-over type or if the pillows are removed and put elsewhere during the day, the cover can be made to lie flat on the bed.

In some cases where quilts are no longer used, 'night spreads' of light-weight materials or even a third sheet, cover and are tucked in with the blankets to give a better appearance to the bed after the bedspread has been removed.

Cots

It is usual in some establishments to have cots available when they are required for children. A cot consists of a mattress on a spring base and to this, sides are attached to prevent the child from falling out. For cots, appropriate sized sheets (often 'remakes' from the linen room), rubber sheets and blankets will be used.

Bed boards

Many guests like a firm bed on which to lie and therefore request a bed board. This is a piece of wood as wide as the bed and almost as long, which is placed between the bed base and the mattress.

Foldaway beds

There are occasions when extra beds are required in rooms and these need to be easily moved and stored away.

Zed-beds have a base of stretched springs which can be folded up, enclosing a thin mattress into a narrow rectangular shape on easy moving castors. They may be surrounded by a valance and the wooden headboard may provide a flat top.

A more comfortable bed is one which folds upright by means of a counter-balanced construction and which can be moved easily on its castors.

Extra beds which remain in the room without taking up space may be stowed away under other beds or may

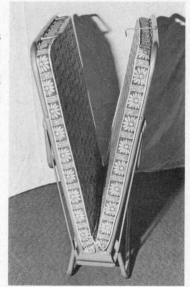

Zed-bed

fold vertically (or horizontally) into the wall to give the impression of a cupboard. There is one type which folds vertically into the wall and

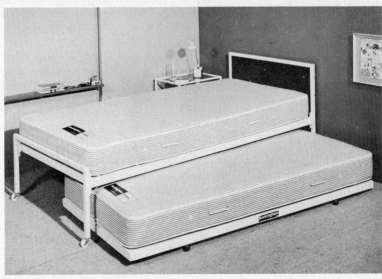

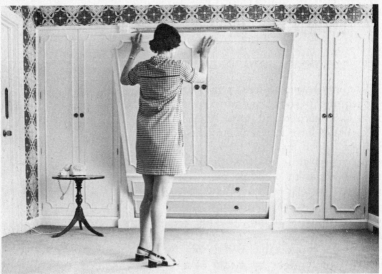

Foldaway beds

part of the underside may be dropped to form a table.

N.B. The term 'bedding' applies to all articles on a bed and should strictly include the launderable linen.

11

Furniture

Furniture in establishments has to stand up to a tremendous amount of wear and tear. People are seldom as careful of other people's property as they are of their own, and the handling of furniture by large numbers of people results in harder use than if one person was using it all the time.

When choosing furniture, several differing requirements should be kept in mind; each piece must be fit for its purpose. Style, comfort, size, serviceability, quality and price are all factors to be considered.

The style of any piece of furniture must tone in with the rest, though it will not necessarily be of similar design. The whole should be in keeping with the style of the room. Dining-room chairs should be chosen with particular tables in mind, but tables and chairs suitable for a canteen will not normally be suitable for a first-class restaurant. It may be an advantage to have a variety of easy chairs in a lounge, some with higher seats, or lower arms, or with wings, but each should be in keeping with its fellows, and none should look as though it had arrived there by accident.

Design and size are closely related to comfort, for inappropriate design or size may interfere with the proper function or the serviceability of an article. The width of the seat and the shape of the back of the chair are important to its comfort: the height of the table and the chair in relation to each other, the height and depth of the wardrobe and the length and width of the bed are other examples. In considering shape and size of pieces of furniture in relation to the body, use is being made of the science of ergonomics. Serviceability will also depend on design; shelves are probably more serviceable in the bedroom than drawers, and 'built-in' furniture can save space, labour, floor and wall coverings.

In large establishments, the quantity of fittings required will probably enable them to be specially designed and ordered (120 chairs is quite an economic number), but many places have to rely on ordinary domestic furniture which is not always suitable for the wear and tear to which it will be subjected. Quality will obviously determine durability, and the mark of the British Standards Institute can be of help when choosing furniture. There is a very wide price range, and most money should normally be spent on those articles which have to withstand

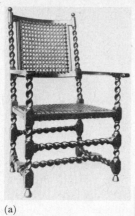

(a)

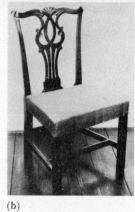

(b)

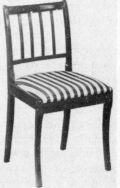

(c)

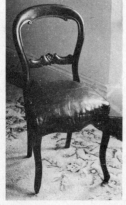

(d)

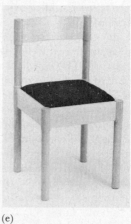

(e)

A variety of chairs (a) early English
(b) Chippendale
(c) Regency
(d) Victorian
(e) modern

greatest wear and tear. The appearance and durability of any piece of furniture will also depend on the material from which it is made, and on its method of construction.

Wood, of course, is the traditional and oldest material for furniture, and pieces dating as far back as 1500 still survive. Anything over a hundred years old is an antique, and beautiful antique pieces may be found in some establishments.

During the 16th and 17th centuries furniture was most frequently made of solid oak or walnut. About the beginning of the 18th century walnut veneers were being used; these were thin slices of wood about 1.5 mm thick (modern veneer may be 0.6–0.8 mm) glued over a carcase of the more common woods of that time e.g. oak, beech, elm, ash or pine. About this period, japanning or lacquering and marquetry (the use of different coloured veneers to form a pattern) also became fashionable.

During the 18th century mahogany became popular and the design of English furniture was influenced by such craftsmen as Chippendale, Hepplewhite, Sheraton and Robert Adam. By the beginning of the 19th century many other woods including amboyna, satinwood and maple were in use as well as the inlaying of metal, generally brass into wood.

The Industrial Revolution brought about the use of machines for the making of furniture and in 1877 William Morris tried to bring about a revival of craftsmanship but machine made furniture had come to stay and the Regency period gave way to the Victorian, and much larger and heavier type of furniture.

Today, with the demand for lighter and more easily moved furniture, there is a very wide choice of woods and the scarcer, more beautiful woods can be used as decorative veneers being glued to woods which are more plentiful, or durable, but which do not have the same eye appeal.

Solid wood is not always the most suitable material for a particular piece, or part of a piece, of furniture, and plywood or laminated wood often meets the requirements of modern furniture better.

Plywood is made by bonding together an odd number of thin slices or plies of wood, 1–2 mm thick, so that the grain of one ply is at right angles to that on either side of it, and since there is an odd number of plies, the grain of the two outside ones will run in the same direction.

Plywood does not warp or twist to the same extent as solid wood, and is equally strong in both directions, whereas solid wood is strongest in the direction of the grain. Plywood is no cheap substitute for solid wood and is frequently used for table tops (7 or 9 ply mahogany) where stability is required, and for curved and shaped parts of furniture which can be preformed, so eliminating much nailing and glueing of parts and enabling stronger and cheaper pieces of furniture to be made.

Solid wood can be bent. Windsor and Bentwood chairs are examples of furniture made of bent pieces of solid wood. Beech is the wood most frequently used but birch, ash and poplar also bend easily.

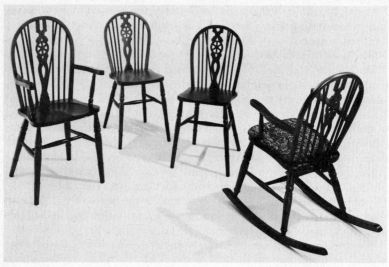

Windsor chairs

Both solid wood and plywood may have decorative veneers on the surface, and if the furniture is to withstand hard wear, there should be some form of lipping, beading or framework, so that the edge of the veneer does not become damaged. Materials such as laminboard, battenboard and blockboard are more stable than plywood (as they consist of softwood strips sandwiched between two veneers); they require no framing and are often used for wardrobe doors.

Laminated wood is also built in layers, but in this case the grain of the layers all run in the same direction; as the strength will be in the direction of the grain, laminated wood is more suitable than plywood for legs and arms of furniture where the greatest strain is in one direction. It may be steam processed so that the arms and legs are made in one curved piece.

Chipboard materials are also used for furniture and these may have an integral melamine facing.

All wood should be guaranteed as properly seasoned, and in this country there should be about 12–14 per cent. moisture, or slightly less where there is central heating. Wood is extremely absorbent. When used for furniture it requires treatment to prevent the absorption of moisture, grease and dirt, in order to make cleaning easier.

There are several protective finishes which may be given to complete the treatment of the wood. It is these finishes which determine the texture of the wood (i.e. whether it has a high gloss, dull gloss or matt appearance), its resistance to abrasion and the ease with which it can be cleaned.

Wood Finishes

Wax. A paste wax polish is rubbed well into the wood; the spirit evaporates and a film of wax is left producing a soft lustre, and it is perhaps one of the most beautiful finishes. A wax finish may be applied to new wood, or stained and filled surfaces; it provides very little protection but it brings out the figure of the wood and imparts a smooth feel. It is maintained by rubbing well when dusting, and polished periodically.

Oil. A mixture of raw linseed oil and white spirit (4:1) is rubbed well into the stained and filled wood. The finish has a slight darkening effect, provides a fair degree of protection, and brings out the natural beauty of the wood. It is frequently used for teak and afromosia, and can be renovated easily. It is maintained by dusting and very occasionally rubbing in boiled linseed oil.

French polish. This is the oldest finish but is fast going out of favour, due to the process being laborious and costly, and not lending itself to mass production. Shellac (a natural resin), dissolved in spirit, is applied to the wood, and by continual rubbing of the hardening shellac and repeated applications a high gloss is obtained. The finish scratches easily and has a very poor resistance to heat, water and alcohol. It is best maintained by dusting and periodically applying a liquid, cream or spray-on wax polish, very sparingly.

Nitrocellulose. This finish is adaptable to all modern production methods, and may range from matt to satin and satin to full gloss. It has good all round functional properties, but its resistance to water and alcohol is only fair. It is maintained by dusting, and in the case of a gloss finish a liquid, cream or spray-on wax polish may be applied periodically.

Acid catalysed (e.g. Melamine). A synthetic resin and a catalyst (required as a hardener) are sprayed or brushed on to the wood which should have been specially stained and filled. The resin is normally of the melamine type and can give a high gloss finish or, if cut back with an abrasive material, a finish resembling the natural wood. Catalyst finishes are the most permanent, heat, water, alcohol and abrasion resistant of all the finishes, but are not as easy to repair or replace. They should be maintained by dusting or wiping with a damp cloth, and a liquid, cream or spray-on wax polish may be applied periodically, if desired, to gloss finishes.

Polyurethane (also a catalyst type). This finish has excellent water and chemical resistance, and the satin finishes have an exceptionally good feel.

Polyester. This finish has a very high gloss and is used principally on radio and television cabinets. It is the most difficult finish to repair.

Wood may be coated with paint when the natural appearance of the wood, i.e. grain, colour, texture, is lost. Paint provides a non-absorbent, easily cleaned finish in a wide range of colours, but it scratches easily and has a poor resistance to heat. It is maintained by dusting, wiping with a damp cloth, or washing when necessary, avoiding the use of strong alkalis and coarse abrasives (see p. 161).

Care and cleaning of wooden furniture
1   Avoid scratching and banging.
2   Wipe up spills as soon as possible.
3   Treat stains as soon as possible (these are often produced as a result of spills not being wiped up quickly enough). (See Chapter 4.)
4   Protect tops of dressing tables, coffee tables, etc., with glass.
5   Examine for woodworm and treat accordingly (see Chapter 14).
6   Clean regularly:

   (*a*) Dust daily, rubbing well to improve appearance.
   (*b*) If necessary, remove any stickiness or fingermarks, with a damp cloth wrung out of warm water and synthetic detergent, or water and vinegar (one tablespoon to a litre of water).
   (*c*) Periodically apply a suitable polish but not to a matt finish or it will lose its appearance and become glossy.

Wicker furniture

This is found in bedrooms and sun lounges of some places and is frequently painted. Unless well maintained it is liable to get out of shape, and pieces of wicker protrude and catch on clothes.
   Cane may be used for the seats and backs of chairs and is occasionally seen on headboards of beds.
   Both wickerwork and cane can become extremely dusty and shabby looking, if not well looked after.

Care and cleaning
1   Examine for broken and protruding pieces of wicker and cane and treat accordingly.
2   Clean regularly:

   (*a*) Dust or use vacuum cleaner attachments daily.

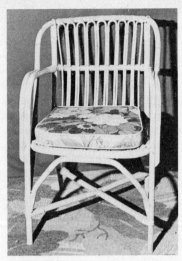

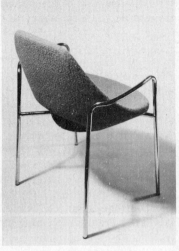

Wicker chair   An example of metal furniture

(*b*) *Wickerwork*: periodically wash, using a cloth or soft nail brush, warm water and synthetic detergent, avoid using a great deal of water. Rinse and dry thoroughly. Polish with a liquid wax furniture polish.

Cane: periodically wash. Rinse with cold salt water and dry thoroughly.

Metals

Metals in the form of iron and steel have been used for many years, for bedsteads and the springs of furniture, but these and many others, owing to their strength and ease of shaping, are being used increasingly in modern furniture.

The metals have great strength and are therefore very suitable for the legs and frames of chairs, and for tables which have tops of such heavy materials as marble or ceramic tiles.

Iron and steel in their various forms, light alloys e.g. aluminium, as well as chromium, brass and copper, are metals frequently used in furniture.

To prevent corrosion many metals require a protective coating and this may be given by anodising, electroplating, or the use of transparent lacquers, plastics, nylon, enamel or other chemical coatings and their appearance may then be maintained by daily dusting or wiping with a damp cloth and washing if necessary.

Mention has been made of the use of marble for the tops of tables. Many tables are used in bars and lounges, where drinks are served, and it should therefore be remembered that acid eats into marble. To protect the marble, the surface may be treated with a catalyst lacquer.

Plastics

Plastics such as the catalyst finishes already mentioned, and synthetic adhesives which have considerable strength and the ability to bond together materials of differing compositions, are used extensively during the making of wooden and other furniture. Nylon and other plastic coatings are given to metal parts to protect them. Laminated and reinforced plastics, however, may form part of the actual piece of furniture.

Laminated plastics are produced as veneers (see Chapter 15) under many trade names, e.g. Formica, and before being converted into furniture parts they require sticking to plywood or similar supporting materials. They are used for table tops, dressing tables, bottoms of drawers, (especially where cosmetics are likely to be spilt) wardrobes and similar pieces of furniture where durability and ease of cleaning are required. Because they have not the 'live' feel of wood, it is possible to compromise, by having the horizontal surfaces on which things may be spilt of laminated plastics, and the vertical surfaces of wood. The appearance of laminated plastics may be maintained by dusting or wiping with a damp cloth. Abrasives should be avoided.

Reinforced plastics used for furniture, are generally of the polyester

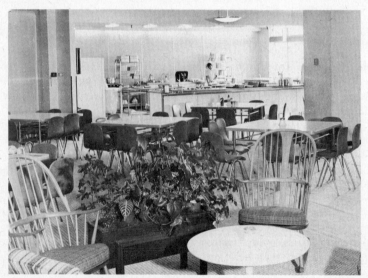

Different types of furniture in a dining room and lounge area

glass fibre type, which can be moulded into seats and backs of chairs, and when used for the shell of upholstered chairs the chairs are much lighter in weight. As laminated plastics, these are durable and very easily cleaned.

Upholstered furniture

The early pieces of furniture were extremely hard to sit on, and to overcome this, some of the ordinary wooden seats and backs of chairs were being padded and covered with fabric by the beginning of the seventeenth century.

Later, it was realised that when padding was to be used, a completely finished piece of furniture was not necessary, and that a framework across which webbing and hessian could be stretched was quite suitable. Layers of suitable stuffing materials, such as tow, sisal, coconut fibre or hair, were then placed on the hessian and held in position by a piece of scrim or calico. So that there should be a reasonable amount of softness, there was next a layer of wadding, prior to the final covering stretched across the whole frame and its stuffing.

The next improvement was to increase the resilience of the upholstered piece of furniture, and this was done by introducing coiled springs between the webbing and the hessian. These added to the size of the article, and many were large and heavy in appearance as well as in weight.

Instead of the coiled springs, tension springs are now often used and the seat consists of a loose piece of foam plastic cut to the shape of the chair and covered with material to match the rest of the upholstery covering. This provides a lighter chair and yet still fully upholstered. Tension springs are also used for easy chairs where the seat and back consist of loose pieces of foam plastic and the wooden frame and arms are not upholstered. These chairs are easier to clean as there are no difficult sides and corners because of the removable seats and backs. In addition, the covers are often fitted with zip fasteners to facilitate their removal for cleaning.

As much of the material and workmanship of upholstered furniture is unseen, it is more difficult to judge its quality than that of cabinet furniture. It is unlikely, however, that a good covering which is well positioned, will hide faulty material or poor workmanship. The covering will, to a great extent, determine the appearance, durability and cost of the piece of furniture. These will be directly related to the quality and suitability of the material from which they are made.

The coverings may be made from textiles, i.e. woven fabrics, hide or plastics. In the case of textiles, their suitability will depend on the type of fibre and yarn, and on the weave used in the production of the fabric. A strong, well twisted fibre, giving a firm yarn which is tightly woven,

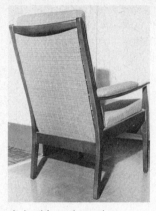

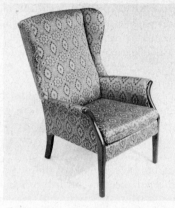

chair with tension springs,
loose seat and back

chair with wooden tip to upholstered
arm and with loose seat

will produce a strong fabric, with abrasion, dirt and snag resistance. The performance of a fabric may be enhanced by the use of stain or soil resistant finishes.

Brocades and damasks of cotton, rayon or synthetic fibres, are smooth fabrics and show soiling more but hold dust less than the rougher textured fabrics such as those made of wool and possibly wool/nylon and wool/Evlan mixture. Although the latter have a warmer appearance they are less slippery and less likely to produce shine on clothes when sat on. Other textured fabrics are the pile ones, velvet, corduroy, moquette, etc. The first two are cut pile fabrics and moquette can be cut or uncut. These may be made of wool, cotton, rayon or synthetic fibres and are hardwearing but hold the dust and may show shading.

The use of synthetic fibres, e.g. nylon, dralon, etc. either alone or in mixtures increases the durability and ease of cleaning of many coverings.

Hide is durable and easily cleaned, but is expensive and must be kept supple to prevent cracking. It is inclined to be cold to the touch and to make clothes shiny when sat on, and for these reasons many pieces of hide furniture have loose fitted seats covered in some woven fabric.

There are many plastic materials available and some resemble hide very closely. They are more easily cleaned, equally hardwearing and less expensive than leather; some have a warmer appearance. They are

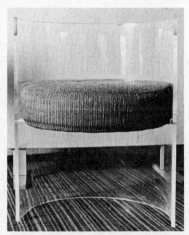

chair in 'perspex' with cushion

normally vinyls, and those with an expandable cotton backing are generally the most suitable. Polyurethane coated fabrics are also being used and these are more comfortable to sit on than many plastic materials as the fabric is not completely non-porous.

Care and cleaning of upholstered furniture

(*a*) *With woven coverings*
1   Watch for signs of wear and deal accordingly.
2   Remove stains as soon as possible (see Chapter 4).
3   Protect, if necessary, with arm covers, chairbacks or loose covers (see Chapter 6).
4   Examine any woodwork for signs of woodworm and treat accordingly (see Chapter 14).
5   If possible, keep out of strong sunlight.
6   If not in use, take precautions against moth.
7   Clean regularly

(i) Remove ash and crumbs daily.
(ii) Brush or use vacuum cleaner attachments frequently, paying particular attention to the corners and sides of the seat.
(iii) Reverse seat cushions to even the wear.
(iv) Dust any showwood parts daily and polish periodically according to finish.
(v) Shampoo periodically as for carpets (see Chapter 8).
(vi) Wash or dry clean any removable covers, when necessary.

(*b*) *With hide coverings*
The care for hide or leather covered furniture is as for woven coverings.
Clean regularly
(i) Dust daily.
(ii) Brush or use vacuum cleaner attachments frequently.
(iii) Periodically polish with good furniture cream to keep supple.
(iv) If slightly soiled—wipe with a soft cloth wrung out of warm water and synthetic detergent. Rinse, dry thoroughly and polish.

(*c*) *With plastic coverings*
The care of plastic covered furniture is as for woven coverings.
Clean regularly
(i) Dust daily and polish showwood parts periodically.
(ii) Brush or use vacuum cleaner attachments if necessary.
(iii) Wipe with cloth wrung out of warm water and synthetic detergent when necessary. Dry thoroughly.

Before considering the individual requirements of certain pieces of

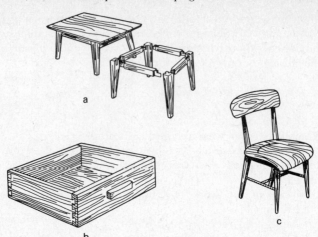

To show methods of joining two pieces of wood:
  (a) mortice and tenon
  (b) dovetail
  (c) dowels

furniture to be used, there are a number of general points which should be considered, when looking for a correctly constructed article.

1   There should be no rough, unfinished edges or surfaces. The backs and the insides should be well made and relatively smooth; the edges of plywood and veneers properly smoothed off, so that they are not liable to be damaged.

2   Joints should be of the right type, tight and well finished. There should be no excess glue round joints. A mortice and tenon joint is used to join two pieces of wood when the tenon is the projection in one piece which fits into the socket in the other.

A dovetail joint is used for jointing drawers, to enable them to withstand constant opening and shutting.

Two pieces of wood such as chair legs, are often joined by means of dowels, round wooden pegs which fit into holes in the two pieces to be joined.

3   Furniture such as dressing tables, wardrobes, tables and chairs, which stands on the floor should be firm and rigid in use.

4   Cantilevered furniture, e.g. dressing tables, luggage racks, etc., should be firmly fixed to the wall to withstand weights that may be put on it.

5   Cupboards and wardrobes should be stable and balanced whether empty or full.

6   Drawers and shelves should be strong enough to carry the necessary articles.

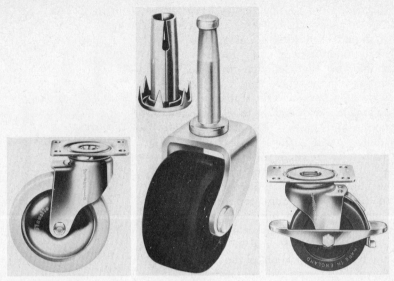

To show a variety of castors

7   Drawers should run smoothly but not slackly, and be fitted with stops.

8   Doors should be well balanced, fit properly and have stays to prevent the doors swinging open too far.

9   Sliding doors should run smoothly.

10   All fastenings should work efficiently; hinges and locks should be substantial but not clumsy. Fastenings may be in the form of locks, plastic or magnetic catches.

11   Handle fittings should be attached in positions most convenient for their use; they should be comfortable to hold and free from sharp edges. Finger grips may be better than handles on drawers.

12   Castors should have no sharp edges to damage the floor and should enable the furniture to be moved easily. (Beds may require a locking device on castors.)

Furniture may be free standing, built-in, fitted or cantilevered. The first is self explanatory while built-in furniture often makes use of part of a wall, and generally cannot be removed without defacement, and fitted furniture is complete in itself but fixed in position. However, the terms 'built-in' and 'fitted' are used loosely to mean the same thing. Cantilevered furniture is fixed on brackets to the wall and hence there are no legs to get in the way of cleaning.

Built-in and fitted furniture save space, as well as wall and possibly floor coverings. They are normally simple in design and they enable the saving of time and labour during cleaning.

Chairs

It should be possible to sit upright easily in any type of chair; the back should be high enough to give support to the whole length of the occupant's back, and the seat should be long and wide enough to relax the thighs and knees. The degree of comfort will depend upon the purpose of the chair, for example in a first-class restaurant the guests are encouraged to have a leisurely meal, so the chairs are more comfortable than those in an establishment where there needs to be a quicker turnover. Comfort will also depend on the size and relative proportions of the chair, the shape of the component parts, the

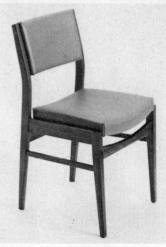

To show space between back and seat for easy cleaning

degree of softness and its relation to other furniture, for example the height of a restaurant chair in relation to the table, a lounge chair in relation to the coffee table.

The depth of a chair seat is generally related to the height of the chair, thus, the lower the chair the greater the depth. An armchair in a lounge, the seat of which is 33–38 cm high, might have a depth of 60–70 cm, whereas a restaurant or writing chair 42–45 cm high would probably have a depth of 42–50 cm. Bar stools are of even greater height and have seats of still less depth. Seat widths are more standard than seat depths, and for an armchair there should be a minimum of 48 cm. With wing chairs the width between the wings is of importance; there should be a minimum width of 56 cm.

Chairs should be strong as many upright ones have to withstand being tilted on their back legs. The legs of dining room chairs should slide easily over the carpet, should not splay out so that they get in the way, and where they are stackable, for example in canteens and banqueting rooms, there may be stops on the legs to prevent scratching.

The covering of a particular chair needs careful consideration, not only in relation to the rest of the décor, but also in relation to the amount and type of soiling it may receive. When restaurant chairs are upholstered, a showwood edge or some wooden grip is useful in preventing constant handling of the upholstery material.

Showwood tips also prevent upholstered arms from getting quite so dirty. A gap between the back and the seat of the chair enables easier cleaning. For comfort this gap should be 20 cm high and the backrest 20 cm, so making the top of the chairback 40 cm above the seat. In the lounge, arm covers and chairbacks may prevent a great deal of soiling on upholstered chairs.

Tables

In restaurants most tables are covered with cloths, so there is no need for decorative tops, but the legs should be of good appearance. For ease of cleaning the top of the table should be covered with a plastic surfaced felt, e.g. Gaylon. When the tables are not covered, they should be of some hygienic, easily cleaned material, e.g. laminated plastic.

For banqueting, easily moved, stackable tables are required, and when these are collapsible there should, as far as possible, be no loose parts, such as wing nuts, which may get lost. Leg frames which take different sized and shaped tops are useful.

The height of the table should be 28–33 cm above the seat of the chair, giving a knee clearance of approximately 18–20 cm when the framing of the table is about 10 cm. The height of the table should therefore be 70–84 cm.

Lounge tables should have a top of some durable material and if of wood may be protected with glass. Coffee tables are approximately 35–50 cm high.

Wardrobes

A minimum of approximately 60 cm of hanging space should be provided in a single wardrobe and 90 cm for a double one, and to prevent the rubbing of shoulders of coats and suits on hangers, the wardrobe should be approximately 56 cm–60 cm deep. In order to take full length dresses a lady's wardrobe should be 175 cm high; a man's wardrobe may be 150 cm with a 25 cm high shelf above for hats. The space above 200 cm is too high to be made use of conveniently, although it is a good idea to take a built-in cupboard or wardrobe to the ceiling, because even if the top is false, a dust trap is avoided.

The hanging rail should be firmly fixed but neither so close to the top nor so thick that it is difficult to put the hangers on it. There should be, if possible, a fitment for folded garments to obviate the necessity for a chest of drawers. It is probably better if the fitment consists of shelves rather than drawers, as these can be cleaned and checked more easily, and the *guest* is less likely to leave articles behind on shelves (see Chapter 13).

It is possible to lease furniture and the leasing contracts for hard furniture and upholstery in leather or expanded vinyl are generally written over a 5-year lease period. For soft furnishings the period is shorter, generally 3 years.

Once the particular pieces of furniture have been chosen and bought or leased, their arrangement in the room is of importance. The purpose of the room may be such that the furniture arrangement needs to be considered as a whole, e.g. in a bedroom, or there may need to be small groups of furniture, e.g. in a restaurant or lounge, but in all cases the arrangement should give a well balanced, inviting appearance to the room.

12

Interior Decoration (Lighting, Heating, Ventilation, Flowers)

In the past, it was thought that the rooms in an hotel should, as far as possible, give the appearance of 'home from home', but it is now realised that guests, while still wanting to feel at home, expect something different in the way of decoration, and that, colours and designs suitable for the home often have a cold and unfriendly look in the impersonal atmosphere of an hotel. The modern trend for simpler architectural exteriors and simpler designs in furniture and furnishings, lends itself to the use of bolder and brighter colours, and the wise use of colour is but one factor concerned in good decoration.

When choosing colours for any establishment it needs to be remembered that there are certain architectural and psychological aspects of colour; thus colours can substantially alter the apparent size or shape of a room, or add to its warmth, cheerfulness, peace and quiet. Reds, yellows, browns and the darker shades of most colours (i.e. the warm and dark colours) are advancing colours and when used on an end wall may shorten the apparent length of a room, or on a ceiling may lessen its apparent height. Cool colours, pale blues and greens, and lighter shades in general, however, are receding colours and tend to make a small room look larger, but should be avoided in rooms with northerly or easterly aspects because of their cold appearance. While some people have a preference for one colour more than another, it is recognized that many colours have a similar effect on different people; for example, reds, oranges and yellows are found to be warm and stimulating; green is cool and has a soothing and pleasing effect; dark blue can be depressing if used in large areas, while pale blue is fresh and cool; purple has richness, is less depressing than dark blue and less stimulating than red; white can appear hygienic and cold. So, in order that the occupants of a room should not be disturbed by the colours, the function of the room should not be forgotten when the colours are chosen. Thus, the entrance hall should look inviting, the lounge, suites and bedrooms restful, bathrooms clean but not cold (peach and pink may therefore be preferable colours to white); restaurants should have a relaxed atmosphere while bars should be bright and cheerful.

Colours are affected by the amount of light falling on them and so will appear different in areas of light and shade; thus curtains appear darker by day when light enters from beside them, than at night when the light falls on them; pile fabrics show shading according to the direction in which the pile lies; an alcove may appear a different colour from the rest of the wall. The type of surface also affects the colour; a rough surface always appears darker than a smooth, glossy one, because of the many small shadows cast by the roughness. Lastly, colours are affected by their surrounding colours; thus a strong colour reflects on its surroundings and may distort other colours and a large area of bright colour always appears brighter than smaller ones.

In most decorative schemes there will be a main, a contrasting and a neutral colour, and once the main colour is chosen a colour wheel may be used to show related colours to help in the selection of complementary ones, i.e. contrasts. Neutrals, black, white, grey, cream, etc. are not shown on the colour wheel, and can be used with any colour combination.

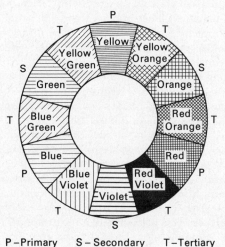

P –Primary   S – Secondary   T –Tertiary

A colour wheel

Because red, yellow and blue cannot be produced by mixing together any other pigments, they are known as primary or fundamental colours. Secondary colours are produced by mixing two primary colours in equal proportions,

thus, red and yellow   = orange
      yellow and blue   = green
      blue and red   = violet

and tertiary colours are produced by mixing a primary colour with a secondary and the exact shade will depend on the proportions,

thus, red and orange = russet, burnt orange, coral, etc.

From the colour wheel such combinations as a triad colour scheme, a complementary, a split complementary or an analogous scheme can be chosen without difficulty.

A triad colour scheme is produced when three primary, three secondary or three tertiary colours are used together, and, for it to be successful, one of the colours should be used in a strong, bright tone in small areas, and the other two should be in softened or greyed tones.

A complementary colour scheme is produced when contrasts are used; the contrast pairs are exactly opposite each other on the wheel, and one should be used in a bright tone for small areas, and the other in greyed tones for larger areas.

A split complementary colour scheme is produced when a particular colour is used with the two on either side of its contrast; it may also include the direct contrast colour, and the same rule applies as for a complementary colour scheme.

An analogous colour scheme is produced when colours which are related are used; they are side by side on the wheel and a contrast colour opposite any one of the group can be used as an accent colour.

Colour is frequently used in conjunction with pattern, and this adds interest to a decorative scheme, but the introduction of pattern is not without its problems, and needs careful consideration. As with colour, pattern can help create the illusion of greater or smaller space; vertical stripes, or any design which tends to move the eye upwards will make a room seem higher, and a narrow room look narrower. Similarly, horizontal lines make a low room look lower and wider. Some patterns have a three dimensional effect giving an appearance of depth and may be useful in a small room.

Too much pattern is disturbing to the eye and creates a 'busy' room, so pattern should be used with restraint, thus a patterned carpet may be used with plain upholstery, patterned curtains with plain walls and vice versa. It is possible to introduce more than one pattern into a scheme, but they should be different in character—a striped and a floral pattern for example—and one pattern should always be dominant. Large patterns can be overpowering in a small room, while small ones may be lost in a large one, so, patterns should be related to the size of the room or object. When choosing patterns, it should be remembered that they appear larger on a small sample than when seen *en masse,* and as far as possible, they should be seen in the position in which they are to be used, carpets lying flat on the floor, wallpaper hanging vertically and curtain materials hanging in folds.

Apart from any interest that patterns may add to the decoration, it should not be overlooked that patterned surfaces do not show marks and soiling as readily as plain ones.

A third factor which contributes to good decoration is texture; in some instances, it takes the place of pattern and in schemes where colour contrasts are not great, texture matters a great deal; thus different tones of gold or yellow may be used without any monotony when the upholstery is velvet, curtains silk and carpet wool.

Much more attention is paid to texture now than formerly and with the wide choice of materials available, variety in texture should not be difficult. In wall coverings alone, texture may vary from the cold, shiny, smooth surface of glass to the warmer, rougher surfaces of grass cloth, hessian and flock paper coverings.

For good decoration, therefore, the need is to try to choose colours, patterns and textures best suited for the particular room, and all three will be introduced into the room by the floor and wall coverings, furniture, furnishings and fittings.

Floorings often outlast other furnishings, so many decorative schemes have to be planned to fit in with the existing floor. Tendency is, where possible, to have fitted carpets throughout the house; this provides only one floor surface to be cleaned and from a decorative point of view, it gives a warm appearance, seems to add space and makes for easier furniture arrangement. A carpet square or a number of small rugs tends to break up a floor area and to reduce room space, and small carpets particularly, separate related furniture groups into distinct units, but, on the other hand they can bring areas of colour, pattern and texture to an otherwise plain floor.

A patterned carpet is normally chosen for large rooms, for rooms with plain walls and/or upholstery, where soiling and staining are to be expected and the floor has to give a good appearance at all times. The design must be chosen carefully so that it is in keeping with the size, style, function and atmosphere of the room.

A plain carpet is particularly suitable for small rooms, for rooms with patterned walls and/or upholstery, and to give an appearance of spaciousness. The colour and tone of the carpet should be such that it unites the whole scheme.

Wall coverings in many decorative schemes are not dominant; they more often than not form a background for the other items. However, this does not mean that they are without colour, pattern or texture, which must, as for everything else, be suitable for the size, style and function of the room. There is probably a wider choice of wall coverings than any other item in the room, when one takes into consideration the different materials, colours, patterns and textures used during their manufacture (see Chapter 9).

Mirrors, framed, unframed or in the form of tiles are sometimes used as wall coverings. Their smooth, shiny surface may be a foil for less smooth surfaces, and due to their reflection they make a room appear larger, increase the light and add to the appearance of a vase of flowers or some similar object. Tinted mirrors are available which give a warmer reflection than the more ordinary silvered ones, and decoration can be increased by designs being etched or engraved on the glass. Careful consideration should be given to the positioning of mirrors on landings, because, although they can be useful in increasing light and the appearance of space, they can be a source of danger to short-sighted and absent minded people.

In many rooms, the windows take up a large part of one wall, and the curtains when drawn at night can then become one wall of the room, and when of a similar colour to the other walls they can produce a very restful effect. The only contrast, in this case, is the texture and the folds of the fabric and, as the continuation of colour increases the sense of space, this treatment is particularly suited to small rooms. Alternatively, the curtains may be chosen to be in contrast to the walls, when they become dominant features in the decorative scheme. Strong pattern, colour and texture add importance to the window and can detract from the size of the room, and it must be remembered, when the windows are large and it is decided to make the curtains the main feature of a room, that the rest of the scheme must be restrained because the area of pattern or colour is large and not broken up in the same way as that of walls and floors.

The proportions of the window and consequently of the room, may be altered by the length of the curtain track in relation to the window, the length of the curtains and where used, by the type and size of the pelmet or valance. For example, a narrow window is given apparent width by the curtain track, and consequently the curtain, extending beyond the window frame; full length curtains may take from the width of a window and make the room appear higher.

Pelmets are generally 1/8-1/6 the height of the curtains and their use as a decorative feature of the room will depend on the material from which they are made, their colour (they may match or contrast with the curtains), and their shape. When there are no pelmets or valances the heading of the curtain is of much greater importance (see Chapter 6).

A bed normally has a headboard which, in many instances, is fixed to the wall behind the bed. From a decorative point of view it should be of a suitable shape, colour and material to fit in with the rest of the furnishings, while from a practical point of view it should withstand frequent cleaning, and be high enough to protect the wall surface when the *guest* sits up in bed.

While floor and wall coverings are important features in the décor, furniture and other furnishings must not be forgotten. For a room to appear comfortable, it must contain furniture that is functional, does not lose the sense of space in a small room, and blends in with the rest of the decoration.

Wood used in furniture has a warm appearance and is normally regarded as a neutral, but certain pieces of furniture, owing to the colour of grain of the wood may be made to stand out from the rest; further

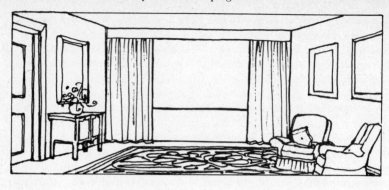

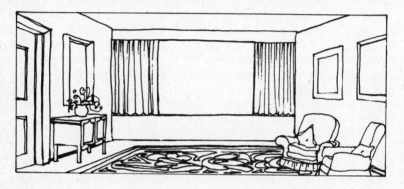

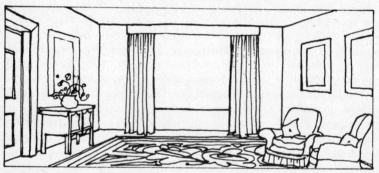

To show the effect of different curtain arrangements

contrasts in colour and texture may be introduced by incorporating metals, glass, marble, plastics and fabrics as part of the furniture. Where the furniture is upholstered or loose covers (including bedspreads) are used, the same care should be taken as for curtains, when choosing the colour and pattern of the fabric. Sometimes the same fabric is used for loose covers as for curtains, and the best effect is probably obtained when only one or two pieces are covered in the same fabric. Textiles are very important to decoration as they provide a large part of the visual appeal and comfort in a room.

A scheme for any room may be softened, or accents of colour can be introduced by the use of pictures, cushions, lamp shades, flowers and other accessories, and even such items as waste paper baskets and ashtrays should be considered with the scheme as a whole.

The size and colouring of any pictures chosen will depend on the wall space available, and the general décor of the individual room. The choice of subject, however, is not as easy, as personal prejudices enter into it, but landscapes and floral paintings probably appeal to the majority of people. Pictures may be sprayed with a plastic which does not alter the colours at all but renders the pictures washable, and enables the glass to be dispensed with, and this may be an advantage as glass has a tendency to cause reflections and get broken. The frame should set off the picture, and be in keeping with the style of the room. Pictures are frequently hung too high; they should normally be about eye level and there should be no cord or wire showing. It is possible to hire pictures and in most hire schemes the pictures are changed about twice a year.

There are some rooms which are used mainly in artificial light, and disappointing results have been obtained when the décor has been planned by daylight. The majority of rooms are, of course, seen in both artificial and daylight, and it must be remembered that parts of the room in shadow during the day, e.g. curtains, may not be so at night, and for good decoration at all times much will depend on the type and positioning of the lights.

It is usual in choosing any decorative scheme to work from the largest to the smallest areas; thus floors, walls and ceilings are considered first, doors, curtains and upholstery next and the smaller areas and accents are decided last.

Lighting

Lighting should be decorative as well as functional; it should contribute to the character and atmosphere of a room, and be adequate for general and particular purposes, without causing glare or appearing flat and dull. To achieve this in any given room, there normally has to be a

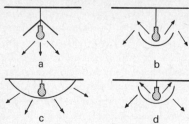

(a) direct lighting　(c) diffused lighting
(b) indirect lighting (d) semi-indirect lighting

balance between direct and indirect, or direct and diffused, lighting systems.

In the case of direct lighting, the fittings throw the light on to surfaces below, generally producing over-bright areas with hard shadows, resulting in glare, and highlights on polished and other smooth surfaces.

For indirect lighting, the fittings are concealed, and the light is thrown on to the ceiling and walls, from where it is reflected into the room. No glare or hard shadows are produced but the lighting tends to have a 'flat' appearance and is very much less economical in use.

When the fittings are completely enclosed or concealed as with ceiling panels or laylights, the light is diffused as it passes through the glass or plastic fitment. Diffused lighting also is glare free and produces a 'flat' appearance. It is possible to have some light passing through a diffusing bowl and some reflected from the ceiling; this is semi-indirect light.

Electric lamps may be filament or fluorescent. Filament lamps are vacuum filled or filled with an inert gas, and generally those above 40 watts are gas filled. The fine filament inside, offers a resistance to the current passing through, and becomes heated to the point of incandescence. The filament may be a single or coiled coil, and the latter having a higher operating temperature gives more light (up to 20 per cent.), and consequently more glare than the same wattage single coil lamp.

Clear lamps give a harsh light and so many are pearl or silica coated, when they give a softer, more diffused light, but even so shades are necessary. The average life of a filament lamp is 1,000 hours (longlife– 2,000 hours) but this may be reduced if the lamp is used in a position other than suspended from its cap. It also happens when there is vibration, wrong voltage or variations in the mains pressure. The cap on the majority of lamps is a bayonet fitting, but lamps of higher than 150 watts may have screw caps. There are tubular shaped filaments or 'architectural' lamps 30 cm–56 cm long.

Filament lamps are low in cost and may be of different sizes and used in many types of fittings, to give direct or diffused light of varying intensities, and are easily replaced. Because they produce sparkle and highlights they are particularly suitable for 'spot' lights, pendant fittings, wall brackets, table and floor standards. Providing the bulb is not coloured, they give a warm light which does not distort colour greatly. They do, however, generate a considerable amount of heat with the consequent soiling and marking of walls, ceilings and shades, and they have poor efficiency and a short life compared with fluorescent lamps.

Fluorescent lamps are vapour filled tubes, coated with fluorescent powders of various colours, and light is produced when ultra violet radiations, resulting from the electric discharge, fall on the fluorescent powders. Different powders have different colours so there are tubes of many colours, and providing care is taken over their choice there need be little, if any, distortion of the surrounding colours. Some tubes have reflectors inside. Hot cathode lamps are most convenient for general lighting purposes as they require a low starting voltage, but cold cathode lamps last much longer, and start instantaneously. Installation of cold cathode lamps, however, is more difficult as they require high voltages.

The average life of a hot cathode fluorescent tube is 5,000 hours, and of a cold cathode 15,000 hours, and this and the fact that their operating temperature is lower—one-fifth lower—than filament lamps, make them very suitable for cornice lights and the lighting of other unget-atable places. Fluorescent lamps give at least three times as much light as filament lamps of equal wattage (coloured lamps even more), so their running costs are lower, but their initial installation cost is higher.

Fluorescent lamps not only vary in wattage but also in length and may be 15 cm–244 cm long. The miniature ones are useful in lighting pictures and direction signs, while the long ones make it possible to light large areas from a single point, and owing to their shape the tubes lend themselves to concealed lighting. They do, however, give diffused lighting, with its 'flat' appearance and it is becoming much more usual when fluorescent lamps are used, to provide textural interest and highlights, by supplementing with filament lamps.

Reflector type incandescent (filament) lamps are being used extensively for feature and decorative lighting. These are usually 100 or 150 watt rating, and have silvered or aluminised inner reflectors which eliminate the need for any form of external light reflectors. Some of these have a pressed glass front of such a construction that they can be used equally well for indoor or outdoor use, provided the lamp holder itself is weatherproof. It is possible to obtain both the spotlight and the floodlight types in both these and the ordinary reflector lamps. Tungsten iodine lamps are the latest type of floodlight unit; in these lamps, there is no blackening of the lamp envelope and hence it can be reduced in size.

Many electric lamps, and in particular filament ones, need to be concealed as much as possible, when the shades and fittings become of great importance to the efficiency of the lighting system, and the decoration of the place in which they are to be used. The filament lamps may be in the form of pendant fittings, wall brackets, table or standard fittings and each one, with its appropriate shade, may be chosen from a very large number of shapes, sizes and materials. Standard lamps should have a firm base and the shade should be in the correct proportion to the base. Where there is any doubt as to size the shade should err on the large side rather than the small. Lengths of flex should be avoided across the floor, over the furniture and under carpets; they are unsightly and may lead to accidents by people tripping over them or by their becoming worn and the consequent danger of fire.

Shades may be of glass, plastic, parchment, fabric or even metal which is generally cellulosed and sometimes perforated. Some materials tend to fade, discolour or become ruined by the heat more than others, but all, in time, become dirty, and not only is the dirt unsightly but it takes from the efficiency of the light. There are instances where the colour of the shade required for the décor casts an unsatisfactory light and so the shade should then be lined. The shade should be pleasing to look at whether lit or unlit. Shades may be dusted or vacuum cleaned with suitable attachments and many may be immersed in warm water and synthetic detergent when special thought should first be given to any trimmings on the shade.

When choosing light fitments consideration should be given to the
    durability and finish of the materials;
    dust collection and ease of cleaning;
    ease of replacement;
    temperature reached after prolonged use;
    weight;
    ease of replacing lamps.

Minimum lighting requirements;

Restaurant	7 lumens/929 cm²
Bathroom	10 lumens/929 cm²
Stairs	10 lumens/929 cm²
General Offices	15–20 lumens/929 cm²
Casual reading	15 lumens/929 cm²
Sustained reading	30 lumens/929 cm²

The entrance hall to any establishment should look inviting and the lighting should be in keeping with the character and atmosphere of the place. During the daytime an entrance can appear dull and dim after coming in from outside.

In a large area a chandelier or other pendant type fitting may give general lighting, or there may be overall lighting of the ceiling by means of cornice lights when the light will be reflected from the ceiling which should therefore be light coloured. General lighting of the area may also be provided by wall brackets or pelmet type fittings.

If height permits, a false or suspended ceiling may be constructed of various materials, and where of wooden slats the light may come through the gaps between; there may be glass panels inset in the ceiling,

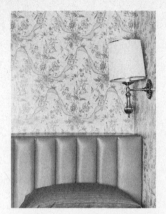

A wall fitting

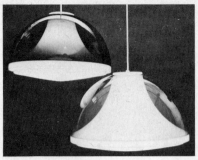

A pendant fitting

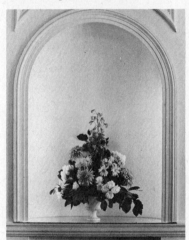

Concealed lighting

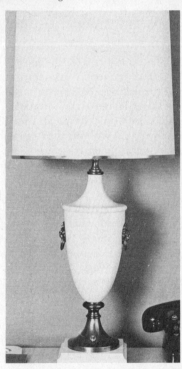

A table lamp

or even holes through which the light passes. An advantage of a false ceiling is that the lamp fittings are concealed (recessed down lights).

Mirrors on the ceiling reflect light and give the impression of greater height and may provide an interesting reflection of the light fittings.

In the entrance hall there should be areas of brighter light to attract *guests'* attention to such places as the reception desk and to enable them to see clearly to sign the register.

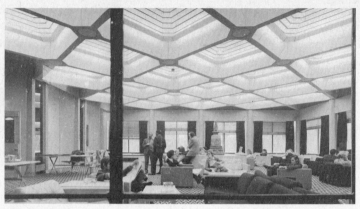

An illuminated ceiling

The atmosphere in the lounge should be one of comfort and restful-ness and as much consideration should be given to the lighting as to the furnishings, bearing in mind that not all parts of the room require the same degree of illumination.

Recessed downlights and wall lights provide some degree of general illumination without the appearance of brightness and may be used as local lights when necessary. In the case of wall lights the light is, however, limited to the perimeter of the room unless there are pillars to which brackets may also be attached. Portable fittings (floor and table standards) are useful and providing there are sufficient sockets available these may be placed in different positions in the room. (Floor sockets, covered when not in use, prevent the trailing of flexes.)

There are many types of places in which food is eaten and the atmo-sphere will vary accordingly. In places where there is a cafeteria service or a quick turnover it is usual for there to be a high degree of illu-mination especially at the counters and tables and in these circumstances fluorescent lamps, pendant fittings or panel lights may be used.

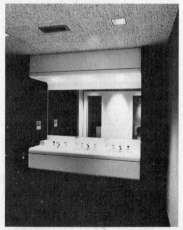

In the restaurant of an hotel, subdued lighting is more usual especially at night when table lamps or even candles may be thought necessary. Higher general lighting is normally used for banquets and luncheons but even so, fluorescent lighting is not often the only source

Recessed lights in a cloakroom with textured ceiling

of light as it provides no highlights, and due consideration should be given to its effect on the colour of food.

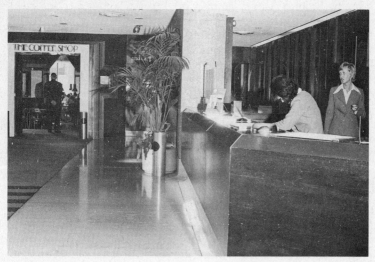

A well-lit reception desk

Subdued lighting may be required in the corridors but gloom should be avoided, and guests should be able to see the room numbers clearly. The space between the light fittings along a corridor should not be greater than 1½ times the distance they are above the floor. Stairs should be well lit to prevent accidents, and lights can be set into the stair itself or along the wall just below the handrail. If the lights are overhead, the fittings should be placed at each end of each flight of stairs.

For safety reasons, corridor and staircase lights should be left on during the night.

Bedrooms do not necessarily require general lighting but there should be adequate light in the different parts of the room. There should be a bedside light for each bed, as well as dressing table light. Bedside lights may be table standards or mounted on the wall, but in each case they should be sufficiently high to light the book being read and not the pillow, top or side of the bed. It is a good idea to have two-way switches to be worked from the door and the bed. In the case of double and twin beds it is kinder to have two lights for reading in bed, each with its own switch, rather than one light only. Dressing table lamps should light the face and not the mirror; two lamps are very suitable or one long fluorescent lamp above the mirror. For a study bedroom or studio room there should be a good light which is adjustable for writing and reading, and

for these purposes an 'Anglepoise'
type of light is very suitable but not
very decorative.

In bathrooms there should be
vapourproof fittings, and the position
of the light by the mirror should be
such that the face is lit adequately.
The switches should be either outside
the room or of the cord type.

There should be secondary or
emergency lighting operated from an
entirely independent emergency
supply, for corridors, staircases,
banqueting rooms and for exit signs.

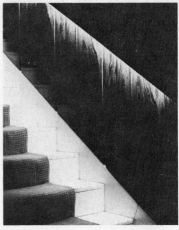

Heating and Ventilation

A staircase lit from below the handrail

The comfort of the human body is
dependent on its being surrounded by moving air of a suitable temperature, humidity and composition, and it is important that these conditions should be produced with the minimum amount of cost and inconvenience, and with some consideration for the design and decoration of
the place.

Individuals vary as to their idea of 'suitable' conditions but it is
generally accepted that there should be a temperature of between 15°–
20°C, a relative humidity of between 40–60 per cent. and not less than
2800 cm³ of fresh air per person per hour. In residential accommodation
for hospital staff the Ministry of Health recommends a background
temperature of 13°C and that the difference be made up with secondary
heating. This is thought to be more economical as rooms are often not
in use.

In areas of establishments covered by the Offices, Shops and Railway
Premises Act 1963 there should be a minimum temperature of 16°C
after the first hour. The occupants of a room contribute continually to
the temperature and humidity of the room, and it is possible that where
there is a large number of people, more changes of air per hour may
be necessary if the occupants are to feel no discomfort. The Ministry
of Health recommends that for nurses' accommodation there should be
1½ changes per hour in a bedroom and 2 changes per hour in a
Common Room.

In most places, bedrooms are ventilated naturally by the use of the
windows, but this may be unsatisfactory in areas where there is a great
deal of external noise, and for such places as bathrooms, cloakrooms,
restaurants and kitchens; some mechanical means may then be necessary to introduce fresh air and/or extract stale air. In the case of internal
bathrooms in London extract ventilation is essential to comform with

by-laws, but there need be no fresh air inlets. Great care should be taken in the siting of the inlets and outlets to prevent draughts, the feeling of stagnation and unsightliness.

In modern establishments, full air conditioning plants are installed when filtered air, at controlled degrees of temperature and relative humidity, enters the individual rooms. Room inlets, mostly in the form of grilles, are generally made of metal, but plaster or wooden ones are available when required to be used from a decorative point of view. Extract gratings remove the air from the room when up to 66 per cent. may be recirculated after being mixed with at least 34 per cent. fresh air and warmed or cooled, dried or moistened as required. Most air conditioning systems work best when the windows in the building are not opened.

In most establishments, there is some form of central heating and the circulating medium may be hot water, steam or warm air produced by the combustion of solid fuel, oil or coal gas, or by the use of electricity. In many systems radiators are required, and these should preferably be placed under the windows when they counteract any downdraughts from the glass, and soiling of the walls is avoided. The modern trend is for the radiator to be enclosed behind a grille; thus difficult and constant cleaning is avoided and the arrangement of furniture is easier. Grilles for warm air should be placed so that they are as inconspicuous as possible. Electric underfloor heating, storage heaters and tubular heaters are other ways of heating the air in a particular room or building.

In public rooms and suites, coal fires aid ventilation, are cheerful and give a pleasing focal point, providing it is not marred by the appearance of the fireplace—(this should be in keeping with the rest of the décor). Coal fires heat rooms unequally and are inadequate for the heating of large rooms without some form of supplementary heating, and this and the fact that they involve a great deal of work, account for their decreasing use, and in most instances their main purpose is as a focal point and not for heating.

In buildings not fully centrally heated or where there is no central heating, other forms of local heating appliances, such as radiant and convector gas or electric fires, will be provided in particular places, for the comfort of the *guests* and staff. These should be chosen for their appearance as well as their efficiency. The efficiency of a radiant electric fire is dependent on the shininess of the reflector and so this must be kept dust free and polished. All open fires, be they solid fuel, gas or electric, must be adequately guarded.

Flowers

In some establishments flowers are used extensively and there may be a large arrangement of flowers in the entrance hall or foyer, flowers in the lounge, restaurant and the suites; in other places there may be only one or two arrangements, but as a rule the *guests* are appreciative of the time and trouble spent on the arrangements, and of the pleasing atmosphere they provide.

The extent to which flowers are used in any place will vary firstly with the degree of luxury, when the arranging of personal flowers, such as buttonholes, sprays and the ordering and despatching of flowers for special occasions, may be a part of the service offered to the guests in hotels, and secondly, with the number of special functions, and thirdly with the house policy.

As the *housekeeper* is responsible for the appearance of most parts of the house, she is naturally concerned with the flowers, but the extent of her responsibility for them will vary from one place to another. She may be solely responsible for the flowers, doing the work herself or delegating it to an assistant; in other cases there may be a part-time florist and if she does not come every day the *housekeeper* will still be responsible for the day to day topping up and the picking over of the flowers. Where a first-class hotel has a full time florist or a florists' shop on the premises, the flowers are not the responsibility of the housekeeper, but even so when guests bring in or have flowers sent to them it is usual for the housekeeper to provide vases and when requested, to arrange the flowers.

The person responsible for the flowers, if non-resident, should live within easy reach of the establishment and the source of supply of the flowers, as personal contact in buying is always best. She needs to enjoy good health as her job is arduous, and she is on her feet a great deal. She should be knowledgeable about flowers as well as proficient at arranging them, and she should be aware of the most suitable ones for certain arrangements, for example, those for restaurant tables or for large displays, of pot plants which are both effective and economical, and of foliage which lasts well. An enterprising florist will use unconventional containers, and will employ things other than flowers to vary the decoration, such as logs of wood, bark, stones, fruit and sometimes even vegetables. The florist requires a flower room in which to work; there should be a sink and running water, containers in which flowers may soak, shelves to accommodate vases and a table or bench as a working surface. There should be a good assortment of vases of different shapes and sizes, wire netting (3.8 cm mesh), plastic coated to prevent rusting, scissors, etc. The smaller items together with dried grasses and all the 'bits and pieces' associated with Christmas decorations are best kept in a drawer or cupboard. The photographs below illustrate the use of varied containers and flower arrangements:

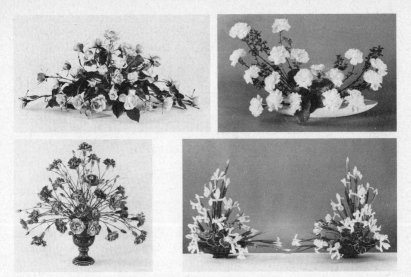

To show various flower arrangements

Artificial flowers

It is true that fresh flowers make for gracious living but they do not last long in smoky and overcrowded atmospheres, such as may exist in busy bars and lounges, and their constant replacement is an expensive item. For these reasons the use of artificial flowers has become more widespread; added to this the quality and design have improved to such an extent, that it is necessary in many cases to touch the flowers, in order to find out whether they are real or not.

Firms under contract will supply the whole arrangement, vase, artificial flowers and foliage, suitable for a particular position. For example, a contract may be made for the provision of one arrangement for the entrance hall to be changed monthly, and the flowers to be consistent with the décor and in keeping with the time of year. Thus there is a saving of time and labour for staff, an avoidance of spills and no space required for a flower room, but it must be emphasised that the provision of artistically arranged artificial flowers is not cheap, though over the year, probably a little cheaper than the use of fresh flowers.

13

Planning Trends (With Special Reference to the Housekeeping Department)

Guests may stay in an establishment for convenience, for pleasure or from necessity and in each case they will require comfort, good food and service, and the provision of these is dependent on there being good planning and organisation throughout the house.

As has been suggested earlier, management relies in many ways on the housekeeping staff for the impression *guests* receive of the establishment, and consequently for their contentment, recommendations and, in the case of hotels, their return in the future. The organisation of the department has already been shown to be of great importance, for if it fails there may be repercussions right through the house. However, in many instances, the impression made on the *guests* can be improved and the work of the staff be made much easier, by careful initial planning of the building, furnishings and fittings.

Alterations and reconstructions in a building can be expensive and difficult operations, and there are places where for one reason or another, they cannot be carried out to any great extent. In these cases the best has to be made of a bad job, and it is unfortunate that sometimes the shortcomings of the establishment's construction and furnishings are given as excuses for the poor or indifferent service offered to the *guests*.

Inconvenience and annoyance to the *guests* and the staff can be caused by:

insufficient or badly placed lifts;
too small service rooms;
badly placed linen chutes or rubbish chutes;
unsightly plumbing or electric wiring;
insufficient lighting and electric sockets;
inconvenient and badly placed furniture and fittings;
unsuitable surfaces for the wear and tear to which they are subjected;
unnecessary dust-traps;
insufficient washing and bathing accommodation.

In many instances, with a little forethought many of these disadvantages could have been overcome, and it is now realised that initial planning, whether for a new or reconstructed building, is of tremendous importance and benefits both the *guests* and the staff. It is for this reason that 'mock ups' and 'trial runs' are being used much more frequently now than formerly. A building should grow from its requirements, so every piece of plant, furniture or fitting should be planned or designed in a functional manner in order that it may accommodate the space available, withstand the abuse it may receive, be comfortable and convenient to the user (*guest* or staff) and be practical in cost.

In order to achieve centralisation of services, for example lifts, emergency exits and chutes for linen and rubbish, due consideration should be given to the shape of a new building. This will obviously be influenced by the space available, and some of the shapes are rectangular, *Y, T,* hollow round and hollow square; in which case the positioning of lifts, fire escapes and chutes is particularly easy.

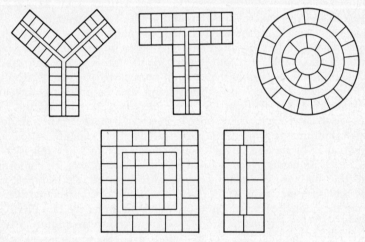

To show Y, T. hollow round, hollow square and rectangular shapes

It is usual for rooms to be on either side of a corridor, so that the maximum number can be provided in a given building, and the window in each room will be in the one outside wall opposite the door. In hotels it may be an advantage to have communicating doors between one room and the next; it is then possible to connect several rooms if required, but on the other hand it may complicate matters when considering the placing of furniture.

The recognised minimum area for a single room is approximately 9 m², a double room 11 m² and for a twin bedded room 13 m²; larger rooms will, of course, mean extra plumbing, lighting, carpeting and furniture. The type of establishment will influence the size of the rooms to some extent and the number of rooms a maid would be expected to service. In a luxury hotel there will be a number of suites; the rooms may be larger than usual; the guests may require more personal service; a maid, therefore, may only service 8–10 rooms, whereas in a less expensive hotel where the tendency is for smaller rooms, a maid may be expected to service 12–15 rooms. In other establishments where little personal service is given, maids may clean many more rooms and so the number of rooms on a floor should be such that it can be divided evenly between the maids, and service rooms should be sited so that the maids do not have to walk long corridors to their sections. Other facilities such as linen chutes, rubbish chutes and ducts for the central suction cleaning system, should also be given careful consideration, so that the maids need to walk as short a distance as possible.

Lifts in many new buildings are fully automatic and travel at a great speed, and there are people who are very nervous of the speed, the confined space and using the lift without an attendant; some have even refused to go to certain hotels owing to the lack of lift attendants.

The corridors should be wide enough to enable the use of trolleys, people to pass comfortably and to prevent any feeling of claustrophobia. Steps can prove a great inconvenience for the use of wheelchairs and trolleys and where possible they should be replaced by ramps. Many corridors have little or no external light, and in order to prevent accidents adequate artificial lighting is necessary throughout the 24 hours; *guests* can then see their way clearly and the room numbers easily. In older buildings, during the day, borrowed light is sometimes used on the corridors by having fanlights over the doors, but when this is the case, *guests* can be disturbed at night by the corridor lights. To conform with local by-laws, secondary lighting must be available in hotels to show up emergency exits. With modern methods of construction there are not the same fire risks in a new building, but under the Fire Precautions Act 1971 fire doors or fire breaks are necessary to confine a fire to one part of the building, and to exclude draughts which might help spread the fire.

Room doors are usually 76 cm to 90 cm wide and they, and the architraves, tend to be simple in design, so giving fewer ledges on which dust may settle; the simple design has the disadvantage of not breaking up a long corridor in the way that more ornate doors and architraves would. This can be overcome, however, to some extent by the use of coloured doors of painted wood or laminated plastic. The outside of the door has the room number on it and in large establishments the number also indicates the floor, e.g. 101 is the first room on the first floor, 201 is the first room on the second floor, and in some hotels the number is also on the inside of the door for the convenience of the guests.

Door locks are of various kinds, and in many establishments it is usual to have a room, a sub-master, a master and a grand master key for the locks (see p. 236). The most satisfactory locks are the mortice ones which fit into a slot in the door frame and are thus concealed from view, and in hotels they should be of the self-locking type; these locks contain a spring bolt which is actuated by a key from outside the room or a handle inside. The keyhole on the outside may actually be in the handle. If a guest requires uninterrupted privacy there is on some locks, a catch which when operated prevents the door being opened by the sub-master or master keys, but the grand master overrides the action of the catch and opens the door, a precaution necessary in case of emergency. Where the lock has no such catch a small bolt is often fixed to the inside of the door and this bolt can be forced without unduly damaging the door. To prevent the surface of the door becoming rubbed by the room key tab, finger plates or metal shields are often placed below the keyholes. Further marking can be prevented by *housekeepers* and maids knocking with their key on the door handle or metal plate instead of on the actual surface of the door.

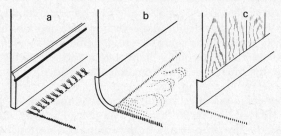

Different skirtings: (a) conventional; (b) metal strip; (c) recessed

Rooms generally have ceilings much lower than previously. During modernisation, it is possible for ceilings to be 'dropped' by making use of plaster boards, acoustic tiles or other materials, thus improving the dimensions of the room, heat and sound insulation.

Walls should be as sound proof as possible to exclude noise from the corridor and the next bedroom. Skirting boards, while essential to prevent damage to the wall, should not present a ledge which needs dusting; they may be slightly recessed, or coved when they may be made of thin metal strips, e.g. anodised aluminium or brass. The coved metal strip enables the edge of the carpet to be cleaned more satisfactorily by an upright vacuum cleaner.

Picture rails are now out of fashion, as with the lower ceilings there is not the need to break the height of the wall, and pictures if any, are normally hung without long cords. Many of the rails in the past held no pictures and were just another ledge which required dusting.

Modern curtain tracks have a better appearance and headings of curtains may be treated in various ways so pelmets are not as necessary as they were. The runners are often plastic and so do not rust, stick or stain the curtain as the older metal ones were inclined to do, unless they were well maintained; in addition the plastic ones make considerably less noise when the curtains are drawn.

Windows should as far as possible be a standard size, as this avoids the need for many spare sets of curtains and sorting curtains of different lengths. The ease with which windows can be cleaned should be given due consideration, and it is an advantage if both sides of the window can be dealt with from inside. Windows may be double glazed to provide either heat or sound insulation; for heat insulation the distance between the two panes of glass should be 0.6 cm while to counteract noise, there should be a space of at least 11 cm, some sound absorbent material at the base between the panes, and one pane should be slightly tilted so that vibration does not get across the gap. It is possible in this way for sound to be reduced 85 per cent. and double glazing in establishments is normally used for sound insulation.

Fireplaces are becoming obsolete and as a result a useful aid to ventilation has been removed, but along with it has gone a source of dust and an entry for birds bringing soot and rubble with them. Most new hotels have an air conditioning plant installed which enables the guest to regulate the filtered, warmed or cooled, and dried or moistened air entering the room and in cases where the windows should not be opened, notices to this effect should be clearly displayed.

In other places, heating is normally by a central heating system which necessitates the use of radiators in the rooms and natural ventilation. The radiators are best placed under the windows and should be enclosed behind a grille to prevent difficult and constant cleaning. Still other places rely on gas or electric fires.

Most new hotels are being built with private bathrooms, but in any establishment, there must be an adequate number of conveniently sited baths and W.C.'s for the number of *guests*, and where there is no private bathroom it is essential in hotels that there should be a wash basin in the bedroom. The wash basin should be sufficiently large, with a mirror, splash back and towel rail, and may be in the form of a vanitory unit (see p. 224).

Lighting in *guests'* rooms should be adequate but not too bright, and it is usual now for there to be several wall, table or standard lamp fittings in a room, rather than centre lights. The lights should be controlled at both the door and the bedhead to prevent a *guest* having to enter the room in darkness, having to get out of bed to turn out the dressing table light for example, and the maid having to put on too much light when calling the *guest*. Bedside lights should be carefully positioned, or be manoeuvrable so that the book is lit and not the top of the *guest's* head; dressing table and wash basin lights should illumine the *guest's* face adequately.

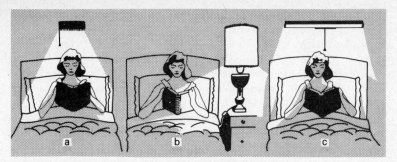

Good bedside lighting by means of: (a) overhead filament lamp
(b) bedside lamp
(c) overhead fluorescent lamp

For appearance and sound insulation, bedrooms should have fitted carpets when there is only one type of floor surface to clean. Where initial cost is a prime consideration, fitted carpets may prove too expensive and so rugs may be laid on cheaper floorings, e.g. linoleum or vinyl, or carpet squares (of varying sizes) may be used with surrounds of the less expensive flooring. Carpet squares and rugs break up a floor surface and tend to make a small room look smaller and there is the added disadvantage that there are two surfaces to be cleaned; they can, however, be turned round to even the wear. A doorstop preferably on the wall is necessary in most rooms to prevent the wall from becoming marked.

Essential pieces of furniture in the *guests'* rooms are the bed, bedside table, dressing table, chair, somewhere to store clothes and maybe a luggage rack, and as more thought is given to the saving of space and the ease with which cleaning can be done, many pieces of furniture are simple in design, built in and have easily cleaned surfaces (see Chapter 11).

Horizontal surfaces should be cantilevered, or reach right down to the floor so that there are no awkward legs in the way of the vacuum cleaner, and all spaces at the tops of wardrobes (above 198 cm is too high for storage) should be enclosed. One unit, the wardrobe, with hanging space on one side, and shelves or open trays on the other, frequently takes the place of the older type of wardrobe and separate chest of drawers. Shelves and open trays are preferable to drawers as *guests* are less likely to leave articles behind on them; they can be more quickly and efficiently cleaned by the maids and checked more easily by the *housekeeper*. The wardrobe should be both long and wide enough, the coathanger rail not too thick and with sufficient space above to enable the hangers to be placed on it easily. Sliding doors save space, but they need to be well maintained and are not as dustproof as hinged ones. In motels where there are many 'one nighters' it is sometimes thought unnecessary to have doors on the wardrobes. Handles, locks and hinges should all be strong enough to withstand the wear and tear to which they are subjected.

Dressing tables are frequently plain, flat surfaces which can be used as writing tables and there should be sufficient knee space. Rounded edges to all corners make for less knocks and rounded insides to the drawers make for easier cleaning, and if the bottoms of the drawers are made of laminated plastic, 'perspex' or some similar material, they need not be lined with paper so saving time. In conjunction with the dressing table there should be a mirror which may be fixed on the wall, or the mirror may be on the underside of the hinged lid of a dressing table fitment.

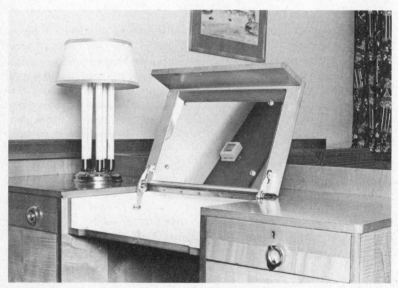

Cantilevered dressing table with mirror on underside of hinged lid

As well as the dressing table mirror, there should be a full length one, which may be fixed to some convenient place on the wall, even fixed to the inside of the door, so that guests may use it to its full advantage, particularly as they are leaving the room.

There should be at least two chairs provided in a single room, an upright one or stool, for the dressing or writing table and a more comfortable one in which the *guest* may relax. Fully upholstered chairs become soiled readily and if without castors, many are too heavy to move easily, consequently chairs with durable frames, webbing and fitted cushioned seats with removable covers, are more practical. However, in hostels and similar places loose seats are often misused.

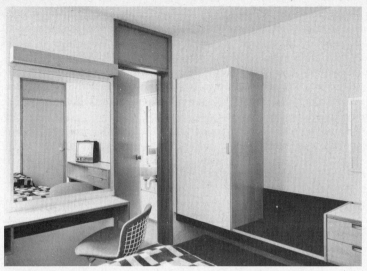

Wardrobe and luggage rack

Luggage racks are usually found in hotels and may be fixed or movable and should be large enough to take a case comfortably, from 60 cm x 46 cm; fixed ones may be cantilevered when they must be strong enough to withstand the weight of heavy cases or someone sitting on them. The surface of wooden luggage racks becomes scratched unless metal strips or a covering of ribbed rubber or similar material is put on them; horizontal stainless steel tubes form a suitable top which is not damaged by the bumping of cases. Where possible some protection should be given to the wall or piece of furniture (often the foot of the

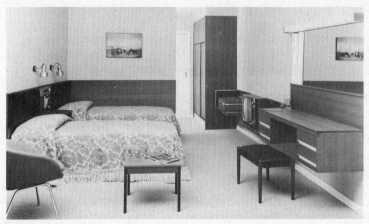

A twin-bedded room

bed) against which the luggage rack rests. Collapsible luggage racks are useful so that when guests have unpacked, the cases and racks may be removed from the room. A strong hook from which a portable wardrobe may be hung is an advantage to the guest who uses this type of luggage, and prevents this being hung from unsuitable places. It is often a problem to know where to put the bedspread when the bed is turned down for the night, and if luggage racks were made with a shelf underneath, this difficulty might be overcome.

The appearance of the room is affected by the size and relative proportions of the various pieces of furniture and fittings already mentioned, but perhaps the article which has the most effect is the bed. In new rooms, the tendency is for beds to be less prominent; they are, therefore, lower than formerly and generally without footboards.

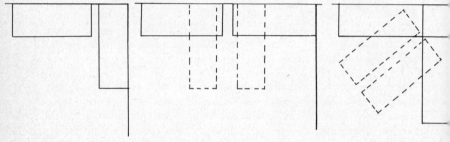

To show different positioning of studio beds

Planning in Hotels

In hotel studio rooms where as much space as possible is required in the centre of the room, twin beds are not placed conventionally side by side, but against the walls, and are used as settees by day.

As the width of a single bed may be 85 cm or 100 cm it is too wide to sit on comfortably, thus it is usual to push part of the bed under a 'back-rest', and the space behind the back-rest often contains the pillows and quilt by day. The back-rest-cum-cupboard (pillow-box) may be the headboard at night and for comfort it should be padded and slant slightly, the widest part covering about 30 cm of the bed. It should, however, not be so close to the covers that difficulty is experienced in pushing the bed under, or in pulling it out. There should be castors or skids on the legs of the beds.

Greater luxury for the hotel guest can be provided by a control panel for light, radio and television switches, within easy reach of the bed, and in many instances this may form part of the headboard, when the latter is fixed to the wall. The newer type of vertical telephone may be fixed

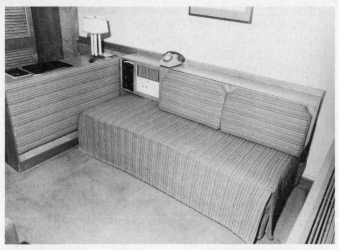

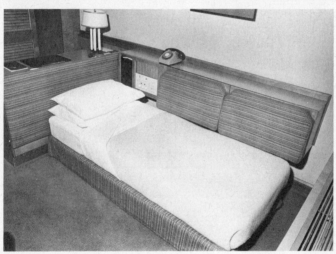

Studio bed by day and night

to the control panel, so saving space on the bedside table and a small light operated from the reception desk may indicate that a message is waiting. In many hotels, guests contact the maid, valet or floor service by telephone, but in others there may be one or more marked bell pushes also on the panel. Attached to the headboard there may be shelves for use as a bedside table and for the storage of telephone books. The bedside table should preferably be cantilevered; it should not be too high but of sufficient size to hold the early morning tea tray comfortably as well as other necessities for the guest.

Breakfast trays can present problems to the guests; either they are lodged precariously on the bedside table, or placed on the bed when their removal requires a feat of agility on the part of the guests wishing to get out of bed. In some hotels the comfort of the guests is aided by providing coffee tables, the top of which can be raised to go over the bed and hold the breakfast tray, and when the meal is finished the table can be pushed to one side.

Television is a feature in many hotel rooms and the set is often placed so that it can be seen from the bed. Tea and coffee making facilities are being provided in more rooms and in some, provisions are made for continental breakfast. Vendors dispensing spirits and other items, fire detectors and alarms and intercom-cum-baby-listener systems may also be found in some hotel rooms. The sales may be automatically recorded at the reception desk, as is the case when the telephone calls are made on the direct dialling system. Iced water is automatically provided in some rooms, while in other hotels there are ice-making machines in the corridors, as well as shoe-cleaning machines. Dumb valets are provided in some hotels to enable the guest to press his own suits.

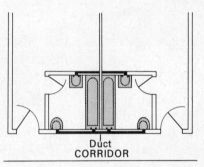

Two bathrooms side by side

A suite usually consists of a bedroom, a private bathroom and a sitting-room and it is an advantage if these rooms can be let separately when required, and with the use of communicating doors it is possible in some hotels to add more rooms. In a suite, meals may be taken in the sitting-room, but more often it is used as a small lounge where drinks are served, so a sideboard with the necessary glasses, is a feature of the room. Relaxed comfort is the predominant factor in these rooms which are close carpeted and have tasteful furnishings and comfortable armchairs. The lighting fitments are decorative and generally include table and standard lamps.

Such articles as waste paper baskets, ashtrays and quite frequently pictures, as well as any articles provided for the convenience of the guests, writing paper, blotters, etc., will also be found in bedrooms or sitting-rooms. In any room the planning of the interior and the arrangement of the furniture and fittings has to be considered from both the functional and decorative angles (see Chapter 12).

With the increased tendency to provide private bathrooms, there has been very much more need for careful planning as the bathrooms are in many instances smaller than formerly (minimum size for a bathroom is approximately 185 cm square with a 168 cm bath, a lavatory basin and W.C.). To cut space still further in some cases there may be a shower in place of a bath.

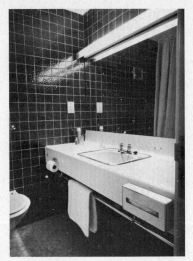

A private bathroom

Bathrooms are frequently internal, and arranged in pairs so that there may be a common duct for drains, water pipes and ventilating shafts, accessible from the corridor.

When bathrooms are internal there must be extract ventilation but building by-laws do not stipulate the introduction of fresh air. Ventilation in a bathroom should always be given very careful consideration as the naked body is very susceptible to draughts and the ventilation shafts can act as sound carriers. In some cases there is an electric fire on the wall or surrounding the light, and in order to avoid the wastage of electricity, switching off the light should automatically turn out the fire, and all switches should be either outside the bathroom or of the cord type.

Bathroom floors should be hygienic and of an easily cleaned material which, if non-porous, sometimes has a sluice hole incorporated; this is a great help when guests let the baths overflow. If floors are carpeted synthetic fibres are preferable to natural or regenerated ones, owing to their low moisture absorbency and quicker drying properties; a loosely laid carpet is an advantage when flooding occurs but ceramic tiles, linoleum or vinyl floorings are much more frequently used.

Baths are generally made of enamelled cast iron or pressed steel although both fibreglass and 'perspex' ones are available; they are obtainable in various colours with soap dishes, grip handles and anti-slip devices sometimes incorporated. Baths are frequently 168 cm to 185 cm long by 70 cm wide, but vary in depth; there is generally about 30 cm of water to the overflow and the latter is approximately 14 cm below the top edge of the bath. There should be ample toe space at the bottom

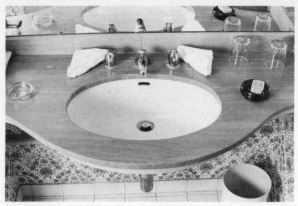

A vanitory unit

of the side panel. Most private bathrooms have showers sited over the bath and these may be thermostatically controlled in order to prevent scalds. The height of the shower, if not movable, should be carefully considered, and a shower screen or a curtain of a suitable length to hang well inside the bath should be provided.

Wash basins are normally made of vitreous china and should be sufficiently large, the most usual size being 56 cm x 40 cm, but there are larger ones of 63 cm x 45 cm; there should be sensible hollows for soap and central or near central taps make cleaning round and under the taps much easier. There should be a mirror above the basin, a razor socket nearby and preferably fluorescent lighting so that the guest's face is well lit. A shelf above the basin is not advisable as it is seldom large enough and there is the danger of articles dropping into the basin and cracking it, but adequate space for toothglass and personal toilet requisites is necessary. A vanitory unit consisting of a flat laminated plastic surface surrounding the wash basin satisfies the need extremely well and has the added advantage that it can be built in and cantilevered. Vanitory units may be used in bedrooms as well as bathrooms.

The W.C. pan is also made of vitreous china and is about 35 cm–40 cm high and 60 cm deep including the cistern (w.w.p.) which is about 50 cm wide; the W.C. pan may be cantilevered and should be of the fully siphonic action type which is not as noisy as the washdown one, is more effective and seldom goes wrong. There is not often room in the new bathrooms for a stool, so the lid of the W.C. may be used as a seat. The cistern may be in the piping duct and accessible from the corridor. Toilet paper holders should be provided, and it is usual for there to be **both tissue and soft paper.**

Bidets, in many countries, are the recognised fourth piece in a bathroom suite and they may be found in private bathrooms in this country. They are made of vitreous china and are about 38 cm high, 36 cm-38 cm wide and project about 58 cm-60 cm from the wall. Their main purpose is for the thorough washing of the anus and genitals, but some people find them useful as foot baths.

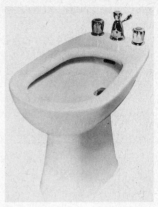

A bidet

Other amenities which should be provided for the guests include towel rails which should be sufficiently far from the wall to allow ample space for the thickness of the towels (when the rails are heated they may be the sole means of heating the bathroom). Drip dry rails over the bath, a hook and a lock on the door should also be provided. Disposable toothglasses may be provided or the toothglasses when cleaned may be put into paper bags. These and the sealing of the W.C. with a paper band have a psychological effect on the guests who consider such practices particularly hygienic.

A telephone in the bathroom can save much irritation and annoyance to guests and it, and the bedroom telephone, may be coloured so that they blend in with the colour scheme of the room.

A ladies' cloakroom (powder room) is provided for the use of guests many of whom will be non-resident and their impression of this room may influence their judgment of the whole hotel. It is usual for there to be several individual W.C.'s, washbasins in the form of vanitory units, large mirrors, coat hanging space and a chair. Where individual towels of either linen or paper are provided there should be a receptacle for the soiled towels and there may be such supplies as tissues, aspirins, feminine towels etc. available. In a first class hotel the décor may be luxurious, e.g. fitted carpet, expensive wall coverings and flattering lighting effect and in such a powder room there will normally be a cloakroom attendant.

Where large functions take place in the hotel e.g. banquets, balls etc. special arrangements may be made for the safekeeping of male and female coats quite apart from the men's cloakroom and the ladies' powder room.

Lounges are provided for guests who wish to spend time in places other than in their bedrooms and the number of these rooms depends on the type of hotel. There are hotels where the lounge is an extension of the foyer and drinks, tea or coffee may be served in a relaxed atmosphere. In city and transient hotels lounges are not normally as numerous as in a resort hotel where in addition to the usual lounge there may be particular rooms set aside for television, reading and writing and even for games.

In a lounge the furnishings will be comfortable and restful and the chairs arranged for guests to be able to converse in small groups. The lighting should give an inviting appearance and chandeliers or lampshades may be an attractive feature.

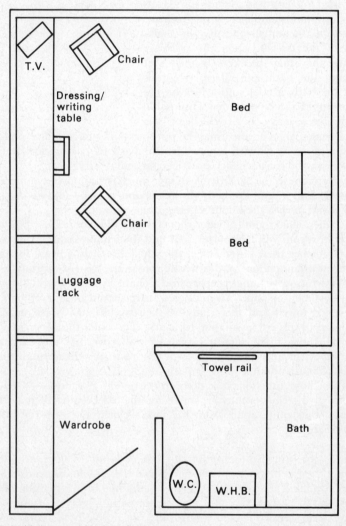

Twin-bedded room with private bathroom

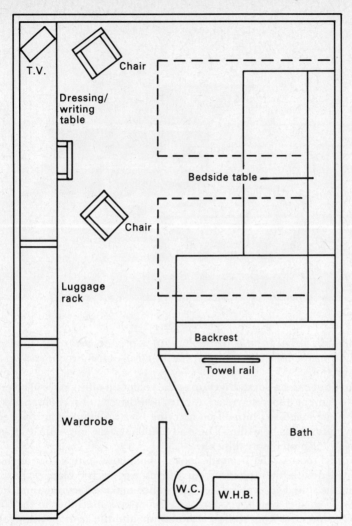

T.V.

Chair

**Dressing/
writing
table**

Bedside table ──────

Chair

**Luggage
rack**

Backrest

Towel rail

Wardrobe

Bath

W.C.

W.H.B.

A studio room showing position of beds by day and night

Motels

Motels are specialised hotels planned for motorists and geared to their requirements. Thus they are situated on or near a main trunk road, and they provide a central catering building and chalet type accommodation, with car parking facilities nearby.

The central building contains the reception office, bars, restaurant and often a coffee shop with a 24-hour service, while the guests' accom-

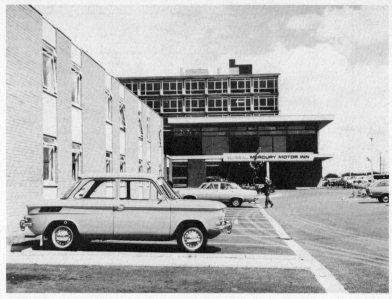

A motel

modation varies from a bedroom with a private bathroom to a suite which may consist of one or more bedrooms, a sitting-room and private bathroom.

In most cases a guest drives up to the reception office, pays in advance for the night and receives a key. He then drives to his room, parks his car nearby and lets himself in, carrying his own luggage and is free to leave as early as he wishes. These advantages to the guest make security within the motel more difficult.

Motel rooms differ from the conventional hotel in that they are often provided with 'do it yourself' equipment, e.g. electric blankets or extra blankets stored in drawers, tea and coffee making facilities, and there may be shoe cleaning, vending and ice-making machines in the corridors, in order to keep staff to a minimum, and the keynote throughout the motel operation is 'convenience' for the guest.

Motor hotels and Post Houses are similar to motels in that they provide the service and facilities thought to be required by the motorist, but the accommodation is not of the chalet type nor is it separate from the central reception and dining block.

Planning in Hostels, University Halls of Residence, Hospitals, Etc.

In modern residential buildings for various types of hostels and halls of residence, the canteen or dining room may be on the premises or it may be some distance away and this will affect the planning.

Usually each floor is similar and is a complete unit for a given number of bedrooms and when there is no dining room on the premises then a utility or communal kitchen/dining area (amenity area) may be provided for a certain number of rooms. This area may be 'open plan' with cooker, refrigerator, sink and draining board as well as a table or tables, and some chairs. If there is a dining room on the premises the utility room usually provides a water boiler or a point for an electric kettle, a work top and maybe a cooker and an ironing board with a fixed electric iron on which there may be a time switch.

Frequently in either case, there are, on the ground floor or in the base-ment, laundry facilities complete with washing machines, driers and irons for the use of all the residents in the building.

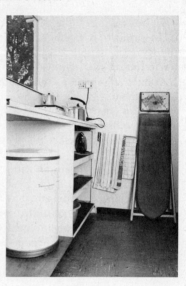

In most places the residents' rooms will be single (though there are places with doubles) and may include wash basins which when enclosed in a cupboard, should have adequate ventilation because of the damp produced from towels, face flannels and possibly washed articles hanging round the basin. On each floor there will be a wash room area which will include bathroom and/or showers, W.C.'s, and if not provided in the bedrooms, wash basins. (N.B. In any case some wash basins should always be provided where there are W.C.'s.)

For example, in one modern hall of residence there are on a floor, 22 study bedrooms each with its own wash basin and the wash room area provides 2 bathrooms, 2 showers, 3 W.C.'s and 2 wash basins.

In another, where there are no wash basins in the study bedrooms, the wash room area provides 2 bathrooms (1 with W.C. and wash basin provided for the use of visitors of the opposite sex), 3 showers, 3 W.C.'s and 6 wash-basins for a floor of approximately 20 students.

The University Grants Committee recommend 1 W.C. and 1 bath for 6 students or 1 shower for 12 and 1 wash basin for 3.

The Ministry of Health recommend for junior hospital staff 1 bath or shower and 1 W.C. for 4–6 people.

The Ministry of Housing recommend for the elderly 1 W.C. for 2 and 1 bath or shower for 4 persons.

The wash room areas should be as conveniently placed as possible for the use of all the residents on a floor. The floorings in these areas are easiest to keep clean and hygienic if they are of an impervious material such as quarry tiles or terrazzo with coved edges. Showers are more economical than baths for water (a shower takes 12½–25 litres and a bath approximately 50 litres) and the heat of the water should be thermostatically controlled. Showers are popular and whereas in hotels they are normally fitted over the bath to save space, in other establishments fewer baths are provided and the showers are sited separately. Opaque curtains of a suitable material are necessary and to prevent accidents there should be a non-slip base to the shower. Soap wells should be provided for both baths and showers; they should be well positioned, allow the water to drain away and be easy to clean.

In hostels and halls of residence for women it is advisable to have incinerators or a 'personnel hygiene service' in the wash room areas for the disposal of soiled sanitary towels. In the first case the towels are burnt and in the second they are treated by a germicidal fluid and the container is on loan and changed regularly in accordance with the requirements of the establishment.

In most modern residential hostels or 'homes', the rooms are bed-sitting rooms or study bedrooms and the latter should incorporate a well lit work table or desk with drawers, an upright chair and shelves for books.

The bed may be 85 cm wide (100 cm is probably too wide for these rooms) and at least 190 cm long with a mattress 'dropped' into the base; this is harder wearing and has a tidier appearance in the room than when the conventional mattress and base are used. Sometimes drawers are fitted in the base for greater storage space. Residents in hostels frequently consider their rooms as their homes and they tend to arrange the furniture to their liking, so with this in mind it may be better to provide beds with headboards rather than to fix headboards to the wall.

The wardrobe should be large enough to allow for bulky winter gear and it should have a lock and key (the usual cupboard above may well prove useful for more permanent storage).

The easy chair should be durable, light weight and easily maintained and a coffee table is often provided. Soft furnishings are kept to a minimum for economy of maintenance; bedspreads are normally of the throw-over type because they probably stand up to the harsh treatment that they are likely to receive better than fitted ones, and so ease maintenance.

Probably the most usual floorings are vinyl or linoleum with bedside rugs, or a fitted cord, tufted or adhesively bonded carpet may be used. Carpeting has the advantage of giving a warmer appearance, better heat and sound insulation and is easier to clean especially if it has been given a stain resistant finish. Wall surfaces are frequently painted.

To avoid nails and Sellotape being used haphazardly on the walls,

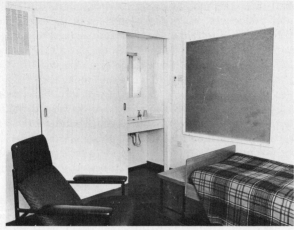

A typical hostel room

a pin board is useful, as well as a firmly fixed towel rail and a good, strong hook on the inside of the door. Because of the inconvenience caused through residents locking themselves out of their rooms, deadlocks of the mortice type rather than the self-locking type of lock on the doors may prove more satisfactory.

In new buildings, the size of a single room varies considerably and may be from approximately 8–10 m². The rooms tend to be longer than they are wide and where students share rooms it may be possible to provide split level working and sleeping areas, so that a student working late is less likely to disturb the other. There should be adequate lighting in the rooms and this will be helped by the provision of sufficient sockets for reading lamps, possibly of the 'Anglepoise' type.

Cork floorings for the corridors have the advantage of being quiet and deadening the sound of footsteps. In new buildings there should be no steps in awkward places, but where they are found, ramps should be arranged for the ease of people in wheelchairs and also for trolleys. The service core, lift well and escape staircase should be as near centrally placed as possible. Wall surfaces on the staircase and corridors may be painted with the multi-colour paints, for hard wear and ease of maintenance but there are other suitable materials.

In addition to the residents' own rooms there will be common rooms and often recreational rooms. In furnishing these rooms consideration should be given to ease of cleaning and the wear and tear to which they may be subjected.

The provision of coin operated telephones, and vending machines of various types is usual in all establishments.

In modern hospitals most of the above points are applicable to the 'homes' and 'residences' where the rooms are of the bed-sitting room type. Vanitory units and fold away beds may be used to get away from the 'bedroom' look and the type of bed where part of the underside lets down as a table, saves space in the room (see Chapter 10). Vinyl wall coverings and vinyl floorings with carpeting make for ease of maintenance.

As far as other areas in the hospitals are concerned there will be tremendous variation in planning; this will depend on the size of the unit and its particular use, e.g. private rooms, wards of varying sizes, day rooms, foyers, waiting rooms, offices, etc. While most parts are kept simple in design and furnishings with the work of the medical and nursing staff, the comfort of the patient, the ease of cleaning and the prevention of cross infection kept in mind, hospitals are being given a more inviting atmosphere than in the past by the use of warmer colours, textured surfaces and more modern designs particularly in the public areas. Thus close carpeting, comfortable furniture and attractive soft furnishings are to be found in foyers, waiting rooms, staff coffee lounges and offices, etc., in some of the modern hospitals. In other cases, PVC tiles, and especially at clinical levels PVC sheet flooring with welded joints and coved skirtings, may be chosen. Where the built in vacuumation system is in use there should be sufficient sockets in order to prevent excessive lengths of hose being used and stored.

Ceilings in the larger areas may be suspended when recessed lights and air diffusers may be contained and acoustic plaster may be used on the walls.

In the larger wards, bathrooms, toilets, sluice rooms, etc., should be as centrally placed as possible to prevent patients and staff having to walk long distances.

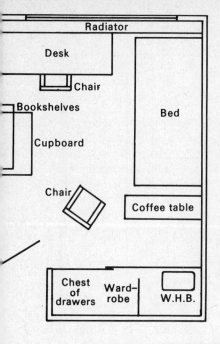

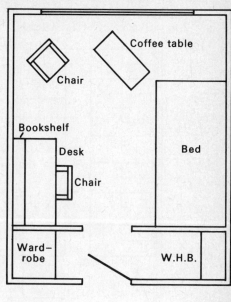

Corridor

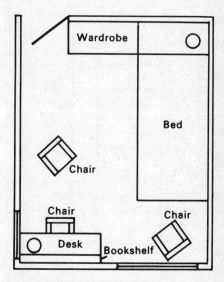

Windows

Anglepoise lamp

Study bedrooms

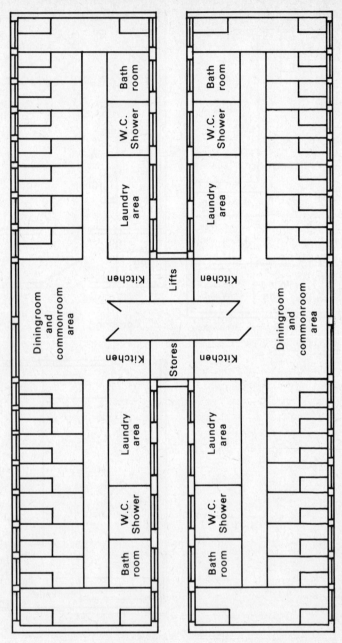

Floor plan of hostels with kitchen dining area

14

Security, First-Aid and Pests

Security is not the prerogative of any one person in an establishment; all staff should be security minded and report anything of a suspicious nature.

Many establishments, e.g. hotels and hospitals, have one or more security officers on their staff to prevent crime and to protect *guests* and their staff from such dangers as theft, fire or assault. A security officer, often an ex-policeman, moves inconspicuously among the guests and is always on the look out for suspicious and undesirable characters. He keeps in touch with other security officers and any information gained is shared among them. He makes clear and concise plans regarding fire precautions, the dealing with bomb threats and the evacuation of the establishment if necessary. He arranges key control and the procedure regarding lost property. He may accompany staff when they go to the bank to pay in money and collect wages and he tries to arrange that the route and the times at which the journey is made should vary to prevent set habits. Other establishments pay a firm to safeguard their money when large sums are being moved from place to place.

Good hall porters, by experience, get to recognise people with a furtive air or remember those who have given trouble in the past. Head hall porters in an hotel may belong to an association through which they exchange information regarding undesirable characters. The time-keeper keeps an eye on the back door and staff comings and goings, and at times may inspect parcels and cases according to house custom. There should be as few unattended doors to the street as possible, and at night all outside doors, except fire doors which only operate from the inside, should be locked and late staff should enter by the front door. Ground floor windows and french windows should have safety catches, and these should be firmly secured at night.

The *housekeeper* and her staff are about the building perhaps more than many other staff and must be aware of the ways in which they can be security minded. If a thief wants to get into a room, it is not difficult for him to gain admittance by telling the maid he has a repair job to do, that he has come to collect some article, that the flowers he is carry-ing are for a certain room or that he has forgotten to collect his key. Therefore, a maid should be instructed to keep a look out for suspicious characters and warned against opening doors for strangers; when such requests are made she must say that she cannot unlock the door, but will fetch the *housekeeper* who should check the name of the guest with reception. Maids should be instructed to lock all doors on leaving a room and to remove all keys left in doors immediately they are seen, and hand them to a *housekeeper* who will return them according to house custom.

Since management has certain responsibilities for the safety of the *guests'* belongings, the proper care of keys is a very important aspect of security. In hotels, there are grand master, master, sub-master and individual room keys. The grand master opens and, in addition, double locks doors against all other keys. In some hotels, this key is held by the duty manager only, while in others, the head housekeeper may also have one. The grand master key is used when access to a room has to be prevented, as in the case of a death or when a guest leaves his belongings and goes away for a night or two, or when a guest does not hand in his key and needs to be seen personally for some special reason. Master keys which open all rooms in the house, are carried by assistant housekeepers while they are on duty and loss of this key may result in dismissal. A sub-master or floor key is carried by a room-maid and it opens all rooms on her floor or section. She collects this key when she starts work and while in her possession, it is attached to a belt round her waist and on no account should it be lent to anyone. She hands it in when she goes off duty and all keys are checked by the duty housekeeper and locked away at night according to house custom. A guest, on being shown to a room, is given a key with a room number and the name of the hotel on the tag. The newer types of locks enable the guest to operate a catch which prevents the door being opened by the sub-master or master keys thus giving the guest a feeling of privacy and prevents them being disturbed by the maid, floorwaiter or housekeeper, etc. The grand master key however, overrides the action of this catch and opens the door, a precaution necessary in the case of an emergency, e.g. illness or accident.

The mastering of locks is necessary but it should be realised that when locks are mastered a certain amount of security is lost and great care should be taken in the allocation of keys to responsible persons emphasising the need for the utmost care in their protection and use at all times. It may be possible to zone rooms so that not all the establishment is in jeopardy should a master key be lost.

Guests are asked to hand in their keys when they go out and the keys are then put on a key board which should be out of view of passers-by as another security precaution.

Most establishments usually have a safe or safe deposit boxes and in hotels notices are displayed asking guests not to leave valuables in their rooms but to have them locked away in the safe. On being admitted to hospital unexpectedly a patient may have with him valuables or a large sum of money which is required to be put into safe keeping. Similarly on the death of a patient there may be articles to be kept until claimed by the next of kin, so suitable security arrangements need to be made in all places. In some establishments residents are advised to take out personal insurance against theft.

It is general that any lost property found in rooms should be handed in to the *housekeeper's* office immediately (or other place according to house custom), and the appropriate details should be entered in a lost property book, after which the articles should be labelled and will usually be kept for a period of six months. Great tact should be exercised in dealing with lost property and it is advocated that guests are not notified of articles found in rooms unless they are still in the building. Precautions need to be taken to ensure that articles are only handed over to the rightful owner and not to any would-be claimant.

The *housekeeper* is responsible for the reporting of faulty window catches etc., and at night should ensure that all french windows and balcony doors are securely locked and that panic bars on fire exit doors are adjusted to enable no entry from outside.

For security reasons the *housekeeper* selects her staff carefully and prospective new members of staff should be asked for the names and addresses of one or two persons to whom reference can be made, and testimonials should not be relied on. In taking up references, it is wise, if possible, to talk on the telephone, rather than to expect former employers to commit themselves on paper.

Fire and *personal injury* are hazards in any establishment and their prevention is another aspect of security. While management is ultimately responsible for the prevention of accidents, the *housekeeper*, along with other heads of departments, should endeavour to see that her staff are safety conscious.

Accidents are costly; there may be serious effects on the injured person; time and materials may be lost; a new employee may need to be trained. Since 1969 employers have been responsible if defective equipment, due to its design or manufacture causes an accident and compulsory insurance against this came into force in 1970 and there may be other insurance and legal costs.

Because poor housekeeping accounts for many accidents and many accidents occur in an establishment's accommodation area (in one survey taken in a group of hotels it was found there were more days lost due to accidents in the housekeeping department than in any other department), the *housekeeper* has a great responsibility in making sure that her staff are aware of the common causes of accidents and the necessary precautions to be taken.

There is a great variety of accidents causing personal injury which may befall *guests* and staff and while they are normally caused through someone's carelessness they are less likely to occur in a clean, uncluttered and well maintained department.

The following are some of the more frequent causes of personal injury which may occur in the housekeeping department.

Falls:
    frayed edges and worn patches of carpet;
    a missing floor tile or uneven floor;
    a missing piece from the nosing of a hard stair;
    slippery floors, especially in conjunction with small mats;
    spills not immediately dealt with;
    trailing flexes from equipment, lamps, television, etc.;
    cleaning equipment left about, buckets, etc.;
    faulty step ladders;
    stools, boxes, etc. used instead of step-ladders;
    poor lighting in corridors and on stairs;
    a step in an unusual place;
    no hand grips on baths.

Cuts and abrasions:
    careless placing of razor blades;
    careless disposal of broken glass;
    careless opening of tins;
    absence of kneeling mats for cleaners.

Burns, scalds and asphyxiation:
    careless lighting of gas equipment;
    careless use of an electric iron;
    absence of fire guards;
    carelessness on the part of smokers;
    newspapers, periodicals, etc. left too near a coal fire;
    faulty electrical equipment;
    misuse of electricity by overloading;
    flexes under rugs and carpets;
    careless positioning of portable heaters;
    covering of heaters and lamps with clothing, towels and similar articles;
    sun's rays striking a concave (shaving) mirror;
    hot water bottles being filled direct from gas or electric hot water heaters;
    careless filling of hot water bottles from kettles;
    too hot water from shower sprays;
    use of certain plastic materials which produce noxious fumes when they catch fire;
    fire stop doors being propped open by wedges and other articles.

Prevention of accidents

Unless precautions are taken accidents may easily occur and the *house-keeper* should therefore see that her staff are made aware of the problems and are instructed in:

the use of correct working methods;
the need for tidiness in their work;
the need for storing things in their right places;
the dangers of floor surfaces being left wet, overpolished, etc.;
the necessity of reporting surfaces and articles in need of repair or replacement;
the advisability of wearing suitable shoes, and clothes which are not constricting.

The staff should be made aware of such dangers as smoking in bed, in such unsafe places as bedding and linen stores and in areas where cleaning polishes and rags etc. are kept; leaving chute doors open, using too strong electric bulbs in lamps, not reporting faulty electrical equipment, sockets, etc. not unplugging electrical appliances e.g. T.V.

The *housekeeper* in addition to training her staff to be aware of the causes of fire and personal injury, should herself make the necessary reports to maintenance and *follow up* these reports.

She should see that provision is made for such things as low wattage lamps for children, hand grips on baths, non-slip mats for use in showers, receptacles for razor blades, good lighting on stairs and corridors (odd steps should be clearly marked or ramps provided). She should see that help is available for the maids when jobs which are heavy or involve much lifting or stretching have to be done.

In the case of fire prevention *the housekeeper* should provide sufficient and suitable ashtrays, suitable waste paper bins, flame proof materials and proper storage for cleaning rags, linen, rubbish and similar articles which may easily catch fire.

It is not always possible to stop fires starting but it should be possible to stop them spreading and endangering life. *Prevention, control* and *escape* are three things which require careful thought when considering the risk of fire. Hotels and similar places have particular problems because guests are often unfamiliar with the layout and spend much of their time in the hotel resting or sleeping.

A fire certificate has been required for those establishments or parts of establishments which come within the Offices, Shops and Railway Premises Act 1963. This Act however did not cover the residential part of hotels and other establishments and the Fire Precautions Act 1971 was introduced to rectify this situation. This Act makes provision for adequate means of escape and related fire precautions in places of public entertainment, recreation and instruction, as well as those establishments providing sleeping accommodation for more than six persons (guests or staff) or where the sleeping accommodation is above the first floor or below the ground floor.

Before a fire certificate is issued the fire authority must be satisfied with such requirements as:

> means of escape and that they can be safely used, e.g. unobstructed escape routes, the use of emergency lighting, clear signs to exits, and fire stop doors,
> fire fighting equipment, specific types in specified areas,
> means of giving warning of a fire,
> staff training,
> fire practices and the appropriate records,
> fire detectors (smoke or heat),
> instructions to guests.

While many of these regulations are more the concern of the manager or maintenance department than the housekeeper, she should have a knowledge of the Fire Precautions Act 1971 and co-operate with management where ever possible.

She should see that her staff are fully aware of the procedure in case of fire. New staff should be given a fire instruction sheet and it may be necessary to have this in several languages. The staff should realise the importance of keeping all escape routes clear, of reporting faulty springs on doors (self closing), exit signs not lit, suspected faulty fire fighting equipment and any movement of equipment, of closing fire stop doors, chute and lift doors and of ensuring that there are instructions to the guest in each room (these too may need to be in several languages).

Fire instructions to the guest should be placed where they are most likely to be seen and more detailed instructions may be placed in maids' service rooms and similar places. Fire alarm and fire exit notices should be illuminated from a source other than the main electricity supply. Automatic fire detection may be by heat or smoke detectors which may be linked to the fire alarm system. In some cases fire stop doors are not kept closed but close automatically when the fire alarm is set off.

In licensed premises and premises offering public entertainment all curtains and similar hangings shall be of such material or so treated and maintained that they will not readily catch fire. All cotton, linen and most rayon fabrics can usually be flame-proofed provided they have not had a special finish. Pure wool, glass fibre and asbestos fabrics are inherently flameproof.

The Treatment of Accidents

Illness, accidents and other emergencies to *guests* and staff unfortunately occur from time to time in any establishment, and in most cases it is the *housekeeper's* responsibility to deal with them. While a *housekeeper* should have a knowledge of first aid, it is essential that she be level-headed and able to take command of a situation, so that it does not become out of hand, and panic, gossip or consternation spread throughout the house. In order to prevent the spread of disquietening facts or gossip, staff should be asked to co-operate and be discreet with the *guests* regarding unfortunate incidents. Inevitably there will be the maid who is anxious to tell the *guests* of an accident or death which occurred in a certain room, and, while it may not worry some *guests*, it will others, and in either case it would be better left unsaid.

A doctor is normally on call, and the *housekeeper* will contact him when necessary, and after his visit she will ensure that his instructions are carried out; in the case of an emergency, 999 may be dialled and an ambulance called. In large establishments, there may be a resident doctor or qualified nurse in attendance, and this relieves the *houskeeeper* of much responsibility. In all establishments there should be accident report forms to be completed giving details concerning any accident which has occurred (e.g. name of person and witnesses, place, date, time and cause of accident, etc.) and in the case of accidents occurring to the staff the accident book required by the Ministry of Health and Social Security must be filled in.

On being told of *guests* or members of staff not being well, the *housekeeper* will visit them, and see to their needs, helping them in whatever way she can, by making them comfortable, allaying any anxiety if possible, and when necessary calling the doctor and following his instructions. In case of notifiable diseases, e.g. smallpox, diphtheria, measles, typhoid fever, scarlet fever, poliomyelitis and whooping cough, the doctor notifies the Medical Officer of Health and if the room needs to be fumigated this will be done with an approved fumigant or by the health authorities.

In order to fumigate a room satisfactorily, windows, ventilators, chimney, keyholes, etc. need to be securely blocked and the chemicals used according to instructions. On leaving the room, the door should be adequately sealed, usually with adhesive paper and the room left undisturbed for the required period of time. Later the room should be well ventilated and thoroughly cleaned.

In the case of a death being reported to the *housekeeper*, she calls the manager and a doctor is called immediately. The central heating or air conditioning should be turned off and to prevent unauthorised persons entering the room, the door is locked until the body is removed. The removal of the body should be done as unobtrusively as possible, and often takes place at night, or some other quiet time when there are few *guests* about. In the case of a suspected suicide, any drinking glass, tablets or vomit must be left for the doctor and/or police as they may be needed as evidence.

First Aid

Besides the First Aid box or cupboard required to be kept in all kitchens, a more comprehensive stock of materials is usually kept in the house-keeping department, and the following are some of the items which might be included:

waterproof adhesive dressings	safety pins
roller bandages	scissors
triangular bandages	antiseptic cream, e.g. Savlon
cotton wool	disinfectant, e.g. Dettol, T.C.P.
gauze	painkiller, e.g. Aspirin, Codeine,
clinical thermometer	Panadol
pair of tweezers	paraffin gauze
eye bath	bicarbonate of soda
pen torch	boracic acid crystals
feeding cup	kaolin
medicine glass	calamine lotion
bedpan and urine bottle	

A *houskeeper* will, of course, only deal with immediate treatment or *first aid*, and will leave special treatment or *second aid* to the doctor.

The following are some of the possible emergencies or illnesses which could occur, and the treatment and remedies given are *first aid* only.

Shock may be caused through an injury giving rise to pain, through haemorrhage or through mental stimulus, such as bad news, and the patient is pale and complains of feeling cold and shivery.

The patient should be laid flat, with all constricting clothing loosened, kept warm by covering with a blanket and given nothing by mouth, except in the case of shock due to mental stimulus when hot, sweet tea may be given.

Fainting may be caused as above, and the loss of blood from the head gives rise to extreme pallor, beads of perspiration and loss of consciousness.

The patient should be laid flat and be prevented from being 'crowded in', so that he gets plenty of air and be treated for shock.

A Heart Attack is due to a clot of blood in the heart and manifests itself by an acute pain in the chest, breathlessness and feeling faint.

The patient should be propped up and on no account moved until the doctor or ambulance arrives.

A Stroke is associated with high blood pressure, and there may or may not be a loss of consciousness, but there is usually some degree of paralysis on one side of the face and body.

The patient should be treated for shock and a doctor called.

Concussion is caused by a blow on the head which may or may not render the patient unconscious. If on questioning later, there is any sign of loss of memory concerning the accident or the time preceding it, then concussion should be suspected.

The patient should be treated for shock and a doctor called.

Diabetes is a disease of the pancreas which prevents the body from burning or oxidising sugar. Many diabetics are treated with insulin which has to be carefully balanced with the diet. If insufficient food is eaten to balance the insulin, the patient starts to perspire and becomes irritable and nervous. Most diabetics carry a diabetic card and sugar for such emergencies, for should this condition be allowed to continue, coma will result.

The patient should be given two lumps of sugar, or a piece of chocolate, at the first sign of insulin shock, and if there is no response, a doctor or ambulance should be called.

Epileptic Fits result in a loss of consciousness and the patient throwing himself about.

The place where the patient has fallen should be cleared of obstacles so that he does not knock himself, and he should be prevented from biting his tongue (and his tongue prevented from falling back) by some suitable object being put between his teeth. The collar should be loosened and the patient left where he is until he recovers.

Convulsions are fits occurring in young children and babies during teething, and frequently herald the onset of the infectious diseases. The child holds its breath, becomes rigid and purple in the face.

The patient should be kept warm by covering with a blanket, or putting into a warm bath and a doctor called.

Asthma results in the patient finding it difficult to breathe and having a feeling of suffocation.

A chronic asthmatic will have had attacks before and may have had drugs prescribed to take during an attack. The patient should be reassured and if necessary, a doctor called.

Poisoning may result from swallowing, inhaling or injecting poisonous substances.

In most cases when poison has been taken by mouth, the patient should be made to vomit by swallowing warm water with salt or mustard in it, and prevented from sleeping until a doctor or ambulance arrives. If the poison is known to be a corrosive, then vomiting should be avoided, and the patient should be taken to hospital as soon as possible. If a person is found unconscious and an empty bottle which contained sleeping tablets is found, an ambulance should be called at once, and the bottle kept as it may be needed as evidence.

Burns are caused by dry heat, hot fat or oil, while a *scald* is caused by moist heat.

There are different degrees of burns and scalds, and for minor ones where the skin is not broken, such as a touch from a hot iron, the affected part should be immersed in cold water.

For more serious burns and scalds, the air should be excluded by covering the affected part with a clean, dry dressing, and applying nothing else because of the risk of infection. The patient should be treated for shock and a doctor or ambulance called.

Burns may also be caused by clothes catching fire when the flames should be smothered by the use of a blanket or heavy coat. The patient should be laid down, treated for shock and if necessary, a doctor or ambulance called.

Electric Shock can be caused by a variety of faults in, and the mishandling of, electrical equipment and may result in burns, shock and even death.

The current should be switched off and artificial respiration applied if necessary. Any burns should be treated and the patient treated for shock and if necessary a doctor or ambulance called.

Cuts and Abrasions may be caused in a great number of ways and may vary considerably, not only in the extent of the damage, but also in the risk of infection as when they are caused as the result of a rusty tin or grit on the ground.

The wound should be cleaned with warm water and antiseptic, and covered with a clean, dry dressing. If bleeding is profuse pressure should be applied:

1   On the wound, if there is no foreign body, e.g. glass or metal, in it.

2   On the pressure point nearest the wound, between the wound and the heart.

The patient should be treated for shock and if necessary, taken to hospital, or a doctor or ambulance called.

Nose Bleeding may be spontaneous or due to a blow, and it is generally more frightening than dangerous.

The patient should be reassured and the nostrils pinched. (The head should not be held back so that the blood is swallowed.) It should be suggested that the nose is not blown for some time after the bleeding has stopped, or the clot may be broken.

Fractures and Sprains are generally caused by a fall giving rise to pain, swelling, and sometimes even bleeding and the bones protruding.

In the case of fractures, movement of the broken bones may cause extensive damage so, in most cases, the person should not be moved until the doctor or ambulance arrives. The patient should be treated for shock, any bleeding arrested and if movement is necessary, the fracture should be immobilised. The patient should be taken to hospital, or a doctor or ambulance called.

A sprain should be bandaged using a crepe bandage, immersed in cold water and the patient treated for shock. If great pain or swelling should occur the patient should be taken to hospital, or a doctor called.

Foreign Body in the Eye may be grit, glass, etc., causing pain.

The injured eye should not be rubbed but bathed with the aid of an eyebath and the nose blown thoroughly. If the object can be seen, it should be possible to try to remove it with the corner of a clean handkerchief. If not removed and the eye is painful, the patient should be taken to the doctor or hospital.

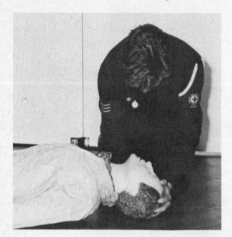 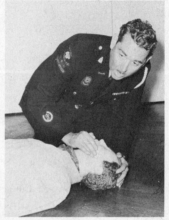

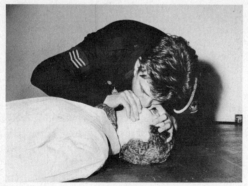

Mouth to mouth or kiss of life method of artificial respiration

Artificial Respiration

The two most usual methods of artificial respiration these days are:

1 Mouth to mouth, or kiss of life.

The patient is laid on his back and his head tilted backwards so that there is a clear passage way to the lungs, by putting a hand under his neck and pulling his chin upwards. His chest is expanded by blowing hard into his mouth (approximately 6 to 10 times a minute), at the same time pinching his nostrils shut, and this treatment is continued until the doctor or ambulance arrives.

2   Holger—Nielsen

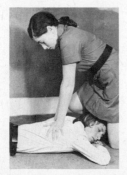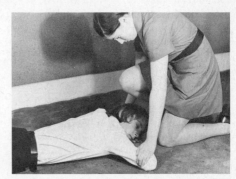

Holger-Nielsen method of artificial respiration

The patient is turned face downwards with his head turned to one side and by kneeling at the patient's head and putting the hands over his shoulder blades, pressure is exerted by slowly rocking forwards (for an adult the pressure should be about 13.6 kg) and as the pressure is released by rocking backwards, the patient's arms are raised by the elbows, to expand his chest, and the process repeated until the doctor or ambulance arrives.

Pests

Moths

Clothes and house moths in the winged state do not feed and therefore during this time they do no damage; their sole purpose is to reproduce themselves and having accomplished this, they die. These moths, of a pale buff colour, are seen flying mainly between June and October; they are relatively small and their wing expanse is rarely more than 2.5 cm. The female moth is normally heavy with eggs and so seldom flies, thus it is the male moth on the wing searching for females which is usually seen; it is rare for either of them to live for longer than a month.

The female lays its eggs on suitable material for the grubs to eat, in some dark, warm place, and one moth may lay up to 200 eggs. The eggs hatch and become grubs (caterpillars) which feed immediately on the material as they move about, and when fully grown they crawl into sheltered places. They stop feeding and spin a cocoon round themselves, become a chrysalis and later emerge as moths to start another life cycle. The entire life cycle (egg–grub–chrysalis–moth) varies from one month to two years depending on the food available, temperature and humidity.

The materials which are attacked by moth (the grubs) are wool, fur, skin and feathers, and those which are immune are rubber, man-made and vegetable fibres. Thus it follows that the articles which need protection from damage by moth are:

1 blankets, bedding and quilts;
2 carpets and underfelts;
3 upholstered furniture and curtains;
4 stuffed animals and birds, i.e. fur and feathers.

Damage by moth most frequently occurs during storage as moths like warmth, darkness and lack of disturbance, and so all articles to be stored should be clean (i.e. vacuum cleaned, brushed or washed), protected by a moth deterrent and inspected frequently. Commonly used moth deterrents are naphthalene, camphor tablets and paradichlorbenzine, whilst insecticides containing pyrethrum are used to kill the pests.

The edges of carpets and upholstered furniture are often attacked by moth, and thus brushing and/or vacuum cleaning with a suitable attachment must be done at frequent intervals. Materials may be treated by a chemical process to render them immune from moth.

Where moth has attacked, for example a blanket, stuffed bird or rolled up piece of carpet, and the articles are found to be full of live grubs, the safest thing is to burn them. Temperatures of 60°C and above will destroy grubs and eggs, and infested articles such as upholstered furniture may be treated by heat providing no harm will come to the articles, or they may be fumigated and in both cases the treatment should be carried out by experts. It should be realised that heat treatment will destroy the moth but not prevent re-infestation.

The common furniture beetle

Wood boring beetles can be likened to moths, in that it is the grub or 'worm' which does the damage to the wood. The common furniture beetle lays about 20–60 eggs in cracks and crevices of unpolished wood, e.g. flooring, panels, backs of wardrobes and chests of drawers. On hatching, the grub eats its way through the wood, and this tunnelling may take from 2–3 years.

In the early spring of the year in which the grub matures, it bores towards the surface of the wood and changes into a pupa which may be compared to a chrysalis. From this pupa emerges the beetle, which bites its way into the open air through an exit hole which is about 0.15 cm in size. The beetles have a very short life (probably 2–3 weeks) during which time they move around by walking or occasionally flying, mating takes place and eggs are laid, often in the old exit holes.

Many pieces of wood have exit holes in them but they may have been successfully treated and are therefore inactive. If, however, small piles of bore-dust are found beneath the holes, these are a sure indication of active 'worms' in the wood, and treatment is necessary, as wood which is infested, in time has innumerable tunnels in it and its strength is badly impaired.

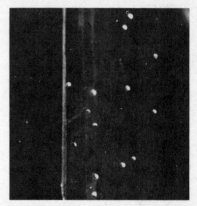

Since the female beetle lays its eggs on unpolished wooden surfaces, the use of shellac, varnish, lacquer or polish acts as a deterrent. To kill woodworm, the exit holes should be sprayed, brushed

To show exit holes of the common furniture beetle

or injected several times with one of the proprietary oil soluble woodworm fluids, e.g. Rentokil or Cuprinol, which may be done by the individual, or experts may be called in to do the job more thoroughly. There are other treatments such as heat and fumigation with poisonous gases but these have disadvantages, do not prevent re-infestation and their use is best left to experts. A badly infested piece of wood is better burnt.

Dry rot

Dry rot is the term used for the decay of timber by a fungus which grows and lives on the wood, and reduces it finally to a dry, crumbling state— hence the name 'dry rot'. It nearly always starts in damp, (more than 20% moisture) unventilated places, behind wood panelling, under floor boards, and spreads by sending out thin root-like strands which creep over brickwork to attack surrounding wood. Once a fungus gets a hold, it produces 'fruit bodies' which are flat pancake-like growths with spore bearing centres. The spores are produced in enormous numbers and are so small that they appear as reddish brown dust which may be blown about very easily and for great distances.

Dry rot can be recognised by its offensive, mouldy smell, by its friable condition and the 'dead' sound when the wood is hit with a hammer. When dry rot occurs it is necessary to find the reason for the dampness of the wood, and the following are some of the more common causes:

1   Slightly leaky joints behind the bath panels, or any faulty plumbing keeping the floor boards damp.

2 Not drying out wet boards under a floor covering such as linoleum.

3 No damp proof course.

4 Ineffective damp proof course through the piling up of earth, coal, sand, etc., against the outside wall.

5 A broken damp proof course.

Having ascertained and cured the cause of the dampness, all rotten wood must be cut away 30 cm–60 cm beyond the infected area and burnt at once—never stored. All brickwork which was near the infected wood, should be sterilised by the use of a blow lamp, and when cool treated with a preservative before repairing with dry, well seasoned timber which should also have been treated with a preservative.

Wet rot

Wet rot is the name given to the fungal decay in timber in very damp situations. The fungus usually involved is the Cellar Fungus and it frequently occurs in buildings, attacking timber that is definitely wet. In view of this, it is commonly found in cellars, roofs and bathrooms, in fact any place where leakage of water is liable to occur. It requires considerably more moisture for development than the Dry Rot Fungus, the optimum moisture content being approximately 40–50 per cent. of the dry weight of the wood.

The fungus causes severe darkening of the wood, which breaks up into small rectangular pieces on drying. There is usually a thin skin of sound wood left on the surface of the timber, but rarely is there much evidence of fungal growth.

Since this fungus requires relatively wet timber and does not possess well developed conducting strands, its eradication is much more simple than in the case of Dry Rot; growth will be checked at once if the timber is thoroughly dried and the source of moisture removed. Badly decayed wood, however, should be cut out and replaced with timber treated with a fungicide, and if there is any possibility of the dampness persisting, then the existing sound timber left *in situ* should also be treated with a suitable preservative.

Fleas, lice and bedbugs

Fleas, lice and bedbugs are insect pests frequently, though not necessarily, associated with dirt. They abound in unhygienic conditions and their entry into clean places may be entirely accidental.

Fleas. There are many different kinds of fleas and each has a preference for one kind of host, e.g. human, cat, dog, vermin, and any of these hosts may introduce fleas into an establishment. Fleas bite their hosts causing annoyance and, in the human, large, red, itching spots on the skin.

Fleas are able to cover considerable distances owing to their jumping powers; they like darkness and warmth, and are capable of laying a large number of eggs, generally in the cracks of floors. Spraying with insecticides is a suitable way of eradicating them.

Lice. Head lice which live in the hair of the head are probably the most common of all lice. They cause intense irritation and suck blood; the eggs, 'nits', which are very numerous, are stuck firmly on to the hairs and cannot be removed by brushing. Lice may be caught from upholstery in trains, by borrowing combs, etc., but are now less frequently found as people have become more hygiene conscious. Frequent brushing, fine combing and when necessary, the use of a special antiseptic are the best remedies.

Bedbugs. Bedbugs may be secreted in second-hand furniture, bedding and books and under the wooden lathes of trunks when luggage has been lying in the holds of ships or in some foreign trains and thus may find their way into any establishment.

Bedbugs are about 0.5 cm long and 0.3 cm wide, reddish brown in colour, and are able to survive sometimes many months without food. They are nocturnal by habit, feed by sucking human blood and deposit their eggs in cracks and crevices of wood work, behind wall paper, etc. The eggs are stuck to these surfaces by a cement-like substance exuded by the bug, and are therefore difficult to brush off.

Bedbugs cover considerable distances although they cannot fly and they give off a very unpleasant smell. Their bites cause considerable irritation and may result in large red patches, with swelling on some people, and the reporting of this condition may well be the first indication that there are bugs in the establishment.

Bugs may be exterminated by spraying with a suitable liquid insecticide, by heat treatment or by fumigation normally carried out by experts. It is important that instructions are followed carefully as some chemicals cause damage to metals and coloured fabrics, and heat may loosen joints of furniture. It must, however, be emphasised that if articles are removed from the room, they should be thoroughly inspected first.

Silverfish. Silverfish are wingless insects, silvery grey in colour and about 1 cm long. The young closely resemble the adults and both are rounded in front and tapered towards the rear. Silverfish require a moist place in which to live and are found in basements, and around pipes, drains, sinks, etc. They leave their hiding places in search of food of a cellulose nature. They feed on starchy foods, paste in wallpaper and books, and may attack clothing made of cotton or rayon, especially if starched. They may be prevented by regular cleaning of cupboards and surroundings to sinks, pipes, etc., and insecticidal powders can be sprinkled where silverfish have been seen.

Rats, mice and cockroaches. Rats, mice and cockroaches are most likely to be found in the kitchen and restaurant/dining room areas, although cockroaches do not necessarily require human food, and will feed on whitewash, hair and books if no other food is available. Hygienic storage and disposal of food and waste and the cleanliness of all areas where food is handled are important points in the prevention of an infestation.

Flies. Flies are of many types and most are attracted to food and food waste. Aerosol sprays are useful in ridding an area of the many varieties that may gain entry to a building.

15

Ceramics, Glass, Plate and Plastics

Ceramics are basically clayware, and during manufacture different types and different proportions of clays, with other ingredients, are mixed to produce the ceramics of the required quality for floor and wall tiles, drain pipes, wash basins, sinks, lavatory pans, vases, cooking utensils, cups and saucers and the like.

The required ingredients are mixed with water to form a liquid mixture which, after various refining processes, becomes sufficiently plastic for the clay to be shaped into hollow or flat ware, either on a potter's wheel or by moulding. The clay body is then fired at a high temperature and changed into hard 'biscuit' ware. After which, a thin film of glaze is applied to the surface of the article, and it is then fired a second time. Decoration when necessary, is applied underglaze or overglaze but gold, because it will not stand up to the high temperature of firing, is generally put on overglaze and thus, of course, it is more liable to be harmed and removed when the article is washed up.

The word 'china' is a broad term which covers all 'clayware' used for crockery and sanitary fittings, and includes glazed and vitrified earthenware, bone china and porcelain.

Glazed earthenware is the ceramic most frequently manufactured in this country. It contains a large amount of ball clay amongst its ingredients, is rather thick, opaque and the glaze is necessary as the clay body is porous.

Vitrified earthenware ('vitreous china') has extra flint added to the clay mixture and has an extra firing when more complete fusion takes place, resulting in heavier, stronger and less easily chipped but more expensive articles.

Bone china contains more china clay (kaolin) and china stone than earthenware and, in addition, calcined bone; the last gives the china its name, makes the clays easier to work and gives the body strength. Bone china is fired at a higher temperature than earthenware, when it becomes almost completely fused and non-porous; it is thin but very strong and more costly.

Porcelain (hard paste china) contains no calcined bone. It is extremely hard, translucent and expensive, and only very small quantities of it are made in this country.

Self-coloured china sometimes has had the clay body dipped in colour and not had the colour incorporated in it, making chips show more easily, although, of course, chipped china should not be used. White china with a simple, easily repeated pattern is probably the most suitable for hotels and other establishments; narrow or broad bands of colour are frequently used for decoration, while badging is a deterrent against pilfering except by the souvenir hunter, but it does entail more careful positioning of the articles on the table.

In order to save the number of articles in use, and storage space, interchangeable pieces, such as jugs for milk and hot water, plates for tea and cheese, make for economy. From a practical point of view, fluted or ridged china is best avoided as it is difficult to clean.

Shallow, broad cups allow liquids to cool very quickly but the taller, narrower ones are more difficult to stack. The depression in the saucer should exactly fit the base of the cup, enabling it to stand firmly. Handles should be tested out with full cups or jugs, and they should be well positioned so that they are comfortable to hold. They should join as near the base as possible to improve rigidity and should not protrude above the top rim. Handles which are moulded on to the clay bodies are called sanitas handles and are less easily broken than those stuck on. They are, however, clumsy looking and the majority of articles have them stuck on, in spite of the fact that they may be more easily broken. Plates should have a rolled edge when chipping of the top of the rim is less likely.

Articles with spouts should be good pourers and jugs should have wide mouths to enable easy cleaning. Teapot lids should have sunken knobs and the lids should be all of the same size for the different sized pots.

Standardisation of china enables breakages to be easily and quickly replaced. The quantity required will depend on peak periods, but 2½ times that required at the peak period is a fair indication of the reserve stock necessary, in addition to the 10 per cent. float of peak number in actual use.

Washing up of china should be done as soon as possible, in order to prevent food sticking to the surface. Preliminary preparation for all washing up should include scraping off food remains, removal of dregs, sorting and arranging the articles in a methodical order.

When using a spray type of washing up machine, careful packing of the articles into the containers is essential, and for all methods of washing up, a suitable detergent should be used, the water for washing and rinsing as hot as possible and the articles left to air dry. When dry, the articles should be checked for mustard, lipstick and tannin stains and dealt with accordingly.

Therefore, whether washing up by hand or machine the articles should be:

scraped of food scraps etc.,

pre-rinsed if possible,

washed in hot water containing detergent, if possible no lower than 60°C,

rinsed in hot water at least 77°C,

drained and air dried.

If necessary, a chemical sterilant may be added to the rinsing water.

With regard to the storage of china, shelves should be checked that they will stand the weight, and piles of plates should not be too large or the bottom ones will crack.

Glass

The main ingredient of glass is sand, which needs to be as free from impurities as possible, and to this, other chemicals are added in proportions depending on the quality or type of glass required.

The carefully measured mixture, known as the batch, is fed into a furnace where it is heated to a very high temperature, 1,300°C or more. From the furnace the molten glass is led away for shaping, after which the glass article has to be very carefully cooled. This is done by annealing; the glass travels on a conveyor belt through an annealing oven, and after the initial reheating, the glass gradually cools as it passes through.

Glass is required for many purposes, tableware, cooking utensils, bottles, vases, lamps, windows, mirrors, etc., and some of these require glass with specific properties.

Soda lime glass is used for ordinary, inexpensive glassware, and the main ingredients are sand, soda ash and limestone. Lead crystal glass is much more attractive to look at; it has brilliance and a fine lustre, and consists of sand, red lead and potash. These ingredients produce a slightly softer glass than soda lime, enabling lead crystal to be cut more easily.

Borosilicate glass is used for ovenware since it is very hard and has special heat resisting properties; it is the borax content which cuts down the rate of expansion when the glass is heated. Borosilicate glass could be used for flame ware but in the United Kingdom flame ware is manufactured from toughened or tempered glass.

Glass required for windows, shelves, etc. is known as flat glass and is made from soda lime glass and is of two main types, sheet and float. Polished plate glass is now largely being replaced by float glass.

Sheet glass is drawn continuously from the molten mass and passed through an annealing tower, after which it can be cut into the required lengths. The thickness of the glass can be varied as the quicker the sheet is drawn off, the thinner the glass will be, and frequently there are flaws in the glass so that a certain amount of distortion occurs. This is, however, becoming less as production methods improve. It is used for ordinary window and picture glass.

Plate glass is made from very refined ingredients, and after being rolled and annealed, is ground and polished. It has, however, been replaced in many instances by float glass which does not require to be ground and polished after annealing. They provide clear, undistorted vision and are used for shop windows, mirrors and protective coverings on furniture. The edges on mirrors are often bevelled, i.e. cut at an angle, while those on shelves are ground and the corners rounded.

Neither sheet nor plate glass will allow the passage of ultra violet light, but it is possible to obtain a special window glass through which ultra violet light will pass.

Obscured glass required for bathrooms, and other places where light but not transparency is required, often has a pattern on one side and this is produced when the molten glass flows from the furnace between embossed rollers.

Wire is sometimes incorporated in the glass during the rolling process, and this is one form of safety glass since the wire prevents the glass falling when broken; for this reason it is used in doors and skylights and as a fire precaution. Other forms of safety glass are laminated and toughened glass. Laminated glass is made in the form of a sandwich of two thin layers of glass with a filling of the vinyl type of plastic in the middle (early types were of celluloid). In this way the glass when broken adheres to the interlayer. Toughened glass is made by subjecting the glass to a temperature just below softening point, and then cooling the surface layers very rapidly. In this way a skin is formed on the glass, and if the glass is broken, it shatters into very small and comparatively harmless fragments. A recent form of safety glass for security purposes incorporates toughening and laminating and is five times stronger.

Hollow glass ware is produced by blowing, moulding or pressing. Most blown glass, today, is made by automatic methods. Cast moulds of wood or iron are often used for shaping the glass, both when it is blown or pressed, and it is sometimes possible to see mould marks on the glass left by the hinges. The moulds may be patterned, giving 'imitation cutting' which is very even, and the cut edges are relatively smooth. Pressing can only be carried out where the top of the container is wider than the bottom, to allow the plunger to be withdrawn. In this method, the molten glass is pressed into all parts of the mould by the plunger.

Cutting of glass is done by hand with abrasive wheels, which rotate at great speed. The cuts at first have a matt surface, but later the article is polished, often by treating with acid, and the cuts on lead crystal glass produce prismatic bodies which give beautiful colours to the glass. Cut full lead crystal glass is expensive, and used for chandeliers, decanters, vases and beautiful table glass. Engraved patterns are made with copper wheels, on to which an abrasive is fed, and these have matt surfaces and are rarely polished. Etching is a further way in which glass can be decorated; in this case the article is coated with a protective wax and the pattern is cut into the wax with a steel needle. On immersing the article in a bath of acid, the acid eats into the unprotected (patterned) areas. This method is a usual way of badging glass which may also be done by engraving, sand blasting or applying an enamel transfer which is fired.

There are many types of drinking glasses in use. They may be plain, fancy, tall, short, stemmed, coloured and some even have handles, but all glasses should be 'en suite' for a well laid table. Certain shapes and sizes are associated with a particular drink, e.g. liqueur, brandy, lager, etc., but those for water, fruit squash, whisky and soda, and others, may be interchangeable.

All glasses should have a firm base and be of a simple design to enable them to be cleaned easily.

Plate

The term 'Plate' is generally accepted as covering all metal table appointments, including cutlery (knives, forks and spoons), flatware and holloware and may be silver plated or of stainless steel. To the manu-facturer, however, 'Plate' applies only to articles electroplated with a precious metal which is invariably pure silver.

Silver is a relatively soft metal which is found naturally in the earth, but more generally in the form of silver salts, from which the metal is extracted. It is a white metal and is unaffected by water, pure air and the majority of foodstuffs. Sterling silver is an alloy containing 92.5 per cent. silver, and the remainder is substantially copper, which is added to harden the silver, and yet not change other properties of the metal. Sterling is obviously more expensive than silver plate and is seldom used in hotels and other places.

Silver plated ware is made from blanks or bodies of a nickel silver, or nickel brass alloy. These are immersed in a complex solution of silver salts, and by means of electrolysis, silver is transferred to the blanks and an electroplated article results. This process gave rise to the symbol 'E.P.N.S.' meaning electroplated nickel silver.

Providing that the blanks are made from a specified nickel silver alloy of the correct thickness, the quality of silver plate is dependent on the electro deposit, which must adhere well, be free from defects and be of a good thickness. As the thickness is not easy to measure, it is expressed as the weight of silver per dozen items of cutlery or flatware, or per single item of holloware in the finished polished condition. Typical deposits for good quality plate would be 45 g per dozen table spoons or forks, 33 g on dessert spoons or forks and 12–15 g on teaspoons, and the silver deposit may be checked at an assay office.

Given reasonable care and usage silver plate will last for many years without any marked change in appearance, but the deposit is relatively soft, and can be scratched or cut by a hard knife blade, or abraded by repeated rubbing in contact with china and glass articles and in either case the base metal will eventually be exposed.

Silver plated ware can be re-plated, but the process is an expensive one as the old deposit has to be stripped off during the preliminary treatment, and if repairs are necessary or desirable at the same time, these will obviously increase the cost. However, good quality silver plate is not cheap in the first instance, and may be excluded from consideration where initial cost is a prime factor; nevertheless, there is no counterpart to silver in terms of appearance and elegance.

The tarnishing of silver is due to the action of compounds of sulphur, present in industrial atmospheres and in certain foodstuffs such as eggs, onion juices, pickles, etc. The tarnish is silver sulphide and varies in colour from yellow, through brown to blue-black, depending upon its thickness. Tarnish is unaffected by simple washing operations but can be removed by immersing the articles in:

1 A hot solution of washing soda, to which a sheet or scraps of aluminium have been added (Polivit method).

2 'Silver Dip' which is a specially compounded liquid chemical mixture and which is almost instantaneous in its action. This liquid will attack stainless steel and it should only be used in a glass, earthenware or plastic container as it is mildly acidic.

With either of the above methods, the articles should be removed immediately the tarnish has disappeared, and thoroughly rinsed, preferably in running hot water, before drying.

In washing up silverware, it is desirable to remove the residues of foodstuffs, prior to immersion in a solution of hot water and detergent. Solid detergents should be completely dissolved, and the articles rinsed in clean hot water and dried whilst hot. Cutlery should always be carefully stacked in appropriate containers, to avoid scratching, and this also applies when washing up by machine.

Other methods of cleaning silver and maintaining or restoring its original bright finish, are available. They involve the use of chemical or mechanical action, or both, by means of:

1 Proprietary preparations, which are complex mixtures in emulsion, paste or powder form and which are rubbed over the articles, buffed off and followed by rinsing and drying. Impregnated polishing cloths may also be used.

2 Metal burnishing, by the use of highly polished steel balls immersed in a solution of water and detergent. The rotation of the container enables the steel balls to roll against the surface of the silver, and restore the bright finish. Holloware articles, in particular, should be suitably positioned in the container to prevent possible damage, and the steel balls should always be kept completely immersed in water, to

prevent them from rusting. Silverware should be rinsed and dried after burnishing.

Research has yielded a preparation to help overcome the problem of silver tarnishing and cleaning. This preparation forms a very thin, colourless, transparent and relatively impervious film, which is chemically bonded to the silver. The film has no odour, taste or other detectable property and in no way affects the appearance of the treated article. The preparation is applied to the silver, and can be used on all silver and plated articles. The film can be broken down by certain acids and alkalis and removed by mechanical action or abrasion, but its tarnish deterrent properties have been fully proved, and articles which have required cleaning every week have retained their original brightness for three months or longer, when treated with this preparation. A similar preparation is available for use on copper and brass.

As silver is a soft metal, and liable to scratching, plated articles should be handled with care. Forks should be kept separately from spoons, carving directly on the surfaces of silver flats should be avoided and dishes should not be allowed to get too hot over naked flames. Although electroplated handles become hot, ebonite or similar alternatives are unsatisfactory as they can prevent the use of the burnishing machine.

There is a tremendous amount of plate used, ranging from vegetable dishes, flats, salts and peppers to spoons and forks and ashtrays and they are usually kept and cared for in the plate room. In addition to those in the restaurant there may be other silver articles in an hotel—in the manager's suite or guests' bedrooms, and the care of these articles will be the responsibility of the housekeeping staff.

Stainless steel owes its corrosion resistance to the effect of the addition of chromium to iron. Knife blades are made from a particularly hard type of stainless steel containing a small percentage of carbon, in addition to the chromium content. Spoons and forks are generally made from a steel containing chromium (18 per cent.) and nickel (8 per cent.) and this alloy cannot be hardened by heat treatment, but is strengthened by cold work, such as pressing and stamping.

Stainless steel is therefore a tough, durable metal and is usually supplied with a mirror polish or satin finish. It can be scratched and it must be remembered that knife edges are appreciably harder than spoons and forks. The washing treatment for stainless steel is similar to that for silver, with adequate rinsing before drying.

The word 'stainless' has been accepted by many people as the complete answer to cleaning problems, but experience in modern catering establishments has shown the need to qualify this assumption. It must be recognised that stainlessness is a relative property, and that stainless steels can be harmed or stained by several substances. For example 'Silver Dip' solutions, chlorine type bleaches, salt-vinegar mixtures and other active agents, are sources of potential attack. In addition, if wet knife blades are left in contact with galvanised or aluminium articles, e.g. draining boards, pans, etc., staining is inevitable. It is brought about by the deposition of a zinc or aluminium corrosion product on the steel, by electrochemical action. The incidence of staining has risen significantly with the increased use of washing up machines. Most detergents have no apparent effect on stainless steels under laboratory test conditions, but there is no doubt that staining can occur when washing up is done by machine. The exact causes and nature of the stains are under investigation, but it would appear that the effect is cumulative with successive washing treatments, and that the stains tend to become 'fixed' and increasingly difficult to remove. In some cases the steel has assumed a dull grey or 'leaden' appearance and an active brushing or scouring action has been necessary to restore the original finish. The general effect can largely be overcome by wiping, and not air drying, after each washing treatment.

Knives may consist of a stainless steel blade securely attached to a handle of other material, or may be a single solid piece of stainless steel. Electroplated handles match the design of the spoons and forks and are generally hard soldered to the blade bolster. Handles made from natural substances, such as wood, bamboo, ivory and horn are often attractive, but may discolour, or be easily damaged in use or in the washing up machine. Synthetic plastics such as xylonite or nylon, are also used but they burn mark easily. Irrespective of materials used, a good quality knife ought to be balanced, i.e. the blade tip should not touch the table when it is laid down.

While there are many designs for cutlery, spoons and forks and many shapes for metal holloware, for large-scale use, patterns should be simple and practical.

Plastics

Plastic to many people conjures up a picture of a beaker, a washing up bowl, a laminated plastic table top or a plastic bag. However, it must not be forgotten that plastics are used for adhesives, protective coatings to metal and wood, sanitary fittings, table ware, fabrics, wall and floor coverings and many other purposes.

Plastics are a group of many substances with similar, though not identical, properties. Thus, they are light in weight, resistant to most chemicals, non-conductors of electricity although they can be made to conduct electricity, combustible but with varying burning characteristics, transparent, translucent or opaque, and thermosetting or thermoplastic. It is perhaps their toughness, although most will scratch with harsh abrasives and sharp articles, and their ease of cleaning which render them particularly useful, and enable them to be put to so many purposes.

Plastic laminates are produced as veneers, and marketed under many trade names, e.g. Formica, Warerite, Duralam, and may be stuck direct to the wall, to plywood or similar supporting material and used as wall panels, counter tops and in the manufacture of furniture. The laminates are manufactured by subjecting layers of paper impregnated with plastic resins such as phenolic and melamine, to great pressure and a high temperature and in some cases now have textured surfaces.

Other plastics used as wall coverings are polystyrene and polyvinyl chloride (PVC) and these may be in the form of tiles, flexible sheets or plastic surfaced papers. Polystyrene and some others, e.g. polyurethane, can be produced as a foam and this, when set, may be used in tile or sheet form on walls or ceilings, to give heat and sound insulation. Still other plastic foams, e.g. those made from polyethylene, polyurethane, etc., have resilience and can be cut into the required sizes for mattresses (see Chapter 10), and into different shapes for upholstered furniture. There is a considerable fire risk with some plastic foams and although these materials can be treated against this hazard, the price is considerably increased.

Polyvinyl chloride has many uses. Plastic floor finishes in tile and sheet form are generally based on it, and PVC may be incorporated with inert fillers, pigments, and plasticisers to give a homogeneous mixture, or it may form a surface layer on some suitable backing. (See Chapter 7.) The durability and ease of cleaning of these floors are dependent on the proportion of PVC present. PVC is also used for soil and waste pipes, electrical conduits, and translucent suspended ceilings.

'Perspex' acrylic sheet and reinforced plastics of the polyester/glass fibre type, are used in the manufacture of furniture, baths, showers and other sanitary fittings. They are very strong, yet light in weight (a 'Perspex' bath weighs about 10 per cent. of the weight of a cast iron one), and in tall, modern buildings where a number of bathrooms may be built one above the other, the weight of the sanitary fittings can be of importance.

Plastics are used in the manufacture of tableware and hardware, and as protective films on metals, wood and natural textile fibres giving increased resistance to abrasion, staining, etc. They can coat fabrics and in the form of a foam sandwich—fabric, foam, skin—they make very satisfactory upholstery coverings. They can also be produced as long filaments and woven into textiles themselves. These synthetic fibres owing to their great strength and poor absorbency are durable, easy to clean and quick to dry (see Chapter 5), and are very useful for carpets, curtains, upholstery, bedding and overalls. For some articles, e.g. blankets, and quilts, the plastic is 'bulked' to render it more fluffy and wool-like.

No doubt more plastics and further uses will be found in the future, but one point has become clear over the past years and that is, that plastics should be considered on their own merits and not as substitutes for natural substances.

Plastics can normally be maintained by dusting, wiping with a damp cloth or washing in hot water and synthetic detergent.

16

The Housekeeper and the Management of her Department

Policy making, that is, the setting out of the objectives and aims of the establishment, is the concern of top management and once a policy has been made a plan should be put into force whereby relevant facts are obtained, information thus received analysed, alternatives considered and the best decision put into effect.

The organising and directing of this decision is normally the work of middle management, and finally there must be some measure of control to evaluate results and to rectify these when they do not come up to standard, and this is supervisory.

Management is concerned with seeing that a job gets done; a manager does not normally perform the tasks himself but he achieves his objectives through people making the best possible use of all his resources.

The *housekeeper* who may be a man or woman, as a line manager is responsible for the efficient and economic running of her department within the aims and objectives as set out by top management. Having ascertained for whom the establishment is intended and the standards to be achieved she has the responsibility of planning and forecasting for her department, organising, leading, directing, controlling and co-ordinating the domestic services under her jurisdiction.

The scope of the *housekeeper's* work varies greatly from place to place and from housekeeper to housekeeper. In the main it is for the organis-ation of the cleaning of the establishment's premises, or such parts as the employing authority dictates (e.g. kitchens, restaurants and dining rooms are not normally the concern of the hotel housekeeper or the hospital domestic superintendent, but they may be of the domestic bursar in hostels), as well as for the management of the staff engaged in the cleaning and servicing of the specified areas. The choice and care of the furnishings also normally come within her scope. (see Chapter 1.) Effective management by the *housekeeper* should lead to the cleanli-ness of the premises, a comfortable and safe environment for the *guests*, the economic running of the department and consideration for the welfare and motivation of the staff.

It is essential for the *housekeeper* to be aware of the aims and object-ives of the establishment as a whole and for her to be informed of and consulted on any policy changes which may affect her department. Costs have risen steeply over the last few years and management has to decide what services it can afford to offer and the best way of providing them. Hotels cannot afford to have empty rooms and some cannot afford to offer the services offered in the past e.g. early morning teas, 'turning down', shoe cleaning, nor can University Halls of Residence afford to have rooms empty during vacations.

A problem arises, not so much perhaps in hotels but in other sectors of the industry, in that top management is often indifferent to the real advantages of good housekeeping. While wanting a clean, safe and comfortable environment, top management may be totally unaware as to how this may be achieved or as to how much it will cost. Objectives and responsibilities are often poorly defined and it is only when housekeeping is an integral part of the whole organisation and the *housekeeper* is armed with the necessary information regarding objectives and responsibilities that she is able to set about managing her department efficiently. She is then able to contribute to the reputation, smooth running and profitability of the establishment.

The *housekeeper* as manager of her department will employ all aspects of managerial activity and while these may be considered separately they are very closely interrelated and all are assisted by good communications.

First, the housekeeper will *plan and forecast* for her department. In this way she will look ahead and try to predict future happenings. She will plan in order that these eventualities are met and that her objectives are reached within the time available. It is possible of course, that however carefully she plans and forecasts circumstances arise over which she has no control.

A good planner thinks on the lines of economy, making the best possible use of time, labour and materials and this will be made easier for the *housekeeper* if she has been consulted at the designing and equipping stage of any new or altered building. Apart from bearing in mind that labour costs account for 90–95% of the total cleaning costs and that cleaning and maintenance costs over a period of about 20 years may equal the initial cost of the building, it should be borne in mind that the planning of areas should be as flexible as possible to enable multipurpose use. Designs should be simple, standardised and planned for easy cleaning but allowances made for change e.g.:

hotel rooms cleared for exhibitions,
suites let as individual bedrooms or meeting rooms,
students' rooms suitable for short term 'lets' during vacations when the status and requirements of the *guests* may be different from the students for whom the hostel was first intended,
hospital flatlets suitable for 1 sister, 2 staff nurses or 4 student nurses as circumstances dictate.

In planning and forecasting for her department the *housekeeper* tries to make the fullest and most efficient use of equipment, space and human effort. She plans what work has to be done, where, when, how and by whom it has to be done having first decided why and whether it has to be done. She thus concerns herself with staffing requirements and becomes acquainted with the whole range of modern cleaning equipment, agents and methods. She should study their advantages and disadvantages and endeavour to bring into use those which make cleaning easier for her staff, save time and are more efficient in producing the final result; in this way she will not only improve working conditions but reduce expenditure and ultimately labour costs.

In setting out to find and implement the most effective use of equipment, space and human effort the *housekeeper* is making use of method study—this is part of Work Study, a 'tool' of management. Work study also includes work measurement which is required to determine the work involved in a job; measurement is made of the time taken to carry out a job under normal circumstances by an average worker. From this a 'standard' time for a defined method may be established. This may help in determining the number of staff required, in determining who is over- or under-employed and in standardising labour costs.

Work study has been applied to various aspects of housekeeping e.g. bedmaking, the planning of the linen room and its work, general cleaning procedures, etc. In a particular investigation it was shown that the distance covered by the maid during bedmaking could be reduced considerably if she stripped the bed more systematically, and did not tuck in the sheets and the blankets until the end of the bedmaking operation.

From other investigations block cleaning rather than a room being completed in one visit have resulted in better working conditions (less fatigue) and better work flow for the staff as well as a saving of time. Individual areas should be planned with a view to the work that will be carried out in these areas and to their relation to the rest of the establishment e.g. maids' service rooms, lifts, linen rooms, etc. Mention has already been made in Chapter 3 of Work Study in connection with the planning of the linen room and the inspection of linen.

Work study should be considered wherever a wastage of time, labour or materials is suspected, e.g.

when delays occur;
equipment lies idle;
work schedules appear unsatisfactory;
overtime appears excessive;
workers are not fully occupied;
rate of absenteeism or accident is high;
excessive movement is suspected;
guests complain of delays, etc.

Sometimes investigations are carried out by trained personnel instead of the *housekeeper* but before any investigation is started a full explanation of the need for Work Study and the way in which it is to be carried out should be given to the staff.

It is not proposed in this book to go into details as to how Work Study is carried out apart from outlining the main steps taken:

1   The job procedure is selected and the problem defined.
2   The present method is recorded by the use of
(a) outline and flow process charts
(b) **flow and string diagrams.**
3   The findings are examined.
4   The improved method is developed.
5   The improved method is installed.
6   Periodic checks are made to ensure the 'improved' method is working satisfactorily.

In any job the best results are obtained after practice. Once the new time and labour saving methods have been acquired the gain will no doubt become apparent, but the change from the 'customary' methods **often takes time and great tact. The staff should be made fully aware** of the new working methods and the reasons for the change. Only with the full co-operation of the staff throughout the investigation is it possible to get a complete picture of the old working methods and to install the improved methods satisfactorily.

Methods used and the time taken on any job will inevitably affect cleaning and the *housekeeper* has to plan a standard of cleanliness. This is almost impossible to measure and while such measurements as dust or bacterial counts can be made they are more suited to specialised purposes, e.g. hospital operating theatres, than for general use.

Other measurements have been based on the number of square metres cleaned per worker, on the annual costs per square metre or other circumstances. These measurements based on statistics, without a full knowledge of the facts on which they are calculated, can be very misleading. Very few areas are identical in

degree and type of soiling,
amount and type of furniture,
furnishings,
obstructions, etc.

and these are but a few of the variables and so the figures can only be 'average'. As a result faulty and expensive decisions may be made. More **often than not, no measurement of cleanliness is taken but the quality** of cleanliness is based on the acceptability or unacceptability of the work.

The *housekeeper* should therefore plan for a standard at the level desired by management, making use of her technical knowledge in defining job procedures, job sequences and frequencies, and work schedules *for her particular establishment*. She may introduce quality supervision when check lists and 'white ragging' can be used in an attempt to compare the work with an ideal standard. The result may be judged as a percentage of the ideal or as fair, good or excellent. (see page 69)

Job procedures and job sequences affect cleaning time as well as cleaning standards and cleaning time is the basis from which staffing requirements stem.

Under standard conditions of equipment, agents, method and personnel a 'standard' time for a job can be found. However, standard conditions seldom exist and although lists of 'standard' time rates have been published by various concerns they should only be used for comparative purposes or as a check list as they cannot take into consideration all the factors which influence the 'standard' time for a particular job in a particular establishment.

Among the factors which will influence the 'standard' time needed for any job are:

the type, age, architectural features of the establishment;
the function of the area;
the maintenance of the area;
the standards to be obtained:
    degree and type of soiling,
    frequency of cleaning,
    type of surface to be cleaned,
    type of service to be rendered;
the amount of traffic and interruptions;
the habits of the occupants;
the accessibility of work areas to service areas;
the availability and type of equipment, supplies, etc.;
the dexterity, motivation and calibre of the employees;
the quality of supervision.

Taking into account the particular circumstances, staffing requirements can be adequately calculated when there is a sound knowledge of average 'standard' time rates needed for any job procedure or sequence. This may be done by totalling all the times for the jobs to give the gross man hours (or minutes) per week (or day). This figure divided by the number of hours (or minutes) to be worked by each member of staff will give the total number of staff required.

Suitable allowances should be made for mid morning or other breaks, preparation and cleaning of equipment, etc. if not built into the 'standard' time. An allowance of 50–60 minutes in a day would not be unusual.

So, assuming daily work takes   4470 mins.
and the cleaners work 8 hours a day   480 mins.
and the allowance for breaks, etc. is   50 mins.
the actual working time per cleaner is
  (480–50)   430 mins.
then, the number of full time staff required is

$$\frac{4470}{430} \; = \; 10.4$$

i.e. 10½ full time employees (F.T.E.) would be required to cover that work.

10% is normally allowed for holidays, sickness, etc.,

so, number of staff = 11½ F.T.E. working 8 hours a day

or 23 4-hourly P.T.E. (part time employees)

When these calculations include time for daily work only, then extra staff will be required to cover periodic cleaning. The calculations are often based on annual hours and in many cases there will be one cleaner required for periodic cleaning to every five for daily work. Thus in the example above 2½ F.T. cleaners would be required for periodic cleaning. However the standard and frequency of periodic cleaning vary greatly and will affect the number of staff required.

There are situations where it may be more beneficial for some work to be done on a cleaning contract rather than by direct labour and the *housekeeper* will have to plan the amount of direct and contract labour required for an economically run department. (Contract Cleaning p. 275)

Where all floors of an establishment are identical and the standard of work throughout is the same per area and per resident or guest, it is not difficult to develop work loads once the staffing requirements and the hours the staff are to work i.e. whether F.T. or P.T., have been established.

  e.g. In an hotel, the room-maids may each service a section of 12 bedrooms with private bathrooms.

     In a students' hostel the cleaners may each be responsible for the cleaning of 20 study bedrooms, washroom block, utility (amenity) room and corridor.

     (If shorter hours are worked obviously each cleaner will be responsible for a smaller section, but more cleaners mean more **money** i.e. overalls, etc.)

On the other hand, where there are different grades of residents and varying types of accommodation the allocation of work is not so simple, if the work load is to be shared equally.

In these cases, a points system may be instituted by which each type of accommodation is given a different point rating (e.g. single room 4 points, double room 5 points, twin bedded room 6 points) and each maid given the same work load according to the point rating of the rooms she services. In other cases a maid may be given an extra room to service for every vacant room in her section, or the number of hours per week for the different types of work or accommodation may be calculated and work allocated accordingly.

e.g. for rooms requiring
      bedmaking and service   3–3½ hrs weekly
      for rooms requiring
      bedmaking but no personal service   2 hrs weekly
      for rooms requiring
      no bedmaking or personal service   1½ hrs weekly
      for vacant rooms (kept ready
      for occupation)   ¼ hrs weekly
      for bathrooms   ½–¾ hrs weekly

In most cleaning operations the *housekeeper* arranges the work on an area assignment basis. The individual maid or cleaner is responsible for one area when the rooms may be cleaned on one visit or in a block. Area assignment may lead to a better pride in the work, a competitive spirit between those working in similar areas, better security and easier supervision as the maid is more easily located.

There are however some cleaning operations planned on a job assignment basis where staff may be working individually or as a team, on a single job throughout the establishment or over a wide area. Such jobs may be carpet shampooing, window cleaning, paint washing and floor cleaning. With this system there may be specialisation and so greater efficiency, a saving in training and in equipment, but supervision may not be so easy.

It cannot be over-emphasised that the standards of work which can be achieved in a given time by a given number of employees, will vary greatly from place to place. However, too often, insufficient thought and planning is given to staffing requirements (staff establishments) and as a result the best is not always received from the staff employed. Work has a tendency 'to expand according to the time available for it' and where the housekeeper is making use of more easily cleaned surfaces, newer equipment etc. as they become available, it is possible, without reassessment of the situation, to become overstaffed and for there to be a poor allocation of work load, with consequent discontent amongst the staff. The *housekeeper* must use all the tools of management to deploy her staff economically and efficiently.

Some reasons for the uneconomic running of her department may be:
1 Wastage of labour—too many staff;
                            outdated jobs;

outdated equipment;
little mechanical equipment;
outdated materials;
outdated designs;
stock not being used (money lying idle);
lack of supervision;
lack of planning.

2 Wastage of materials—extravagant use of cleaning agents;
insufficient cleaning of articles;
insufficient care of articles;
wrong methods of cleaning;
extravagant use of heat, light and water.

In putting her plans into operation the *housekeeper organises* the work of her department when personnel and staffing problems take up a great deal of her time. The staffing of the housekeeping department involves recruitment, selection, training and welfare of the staff (these are dealt with in Chapter 1) as well as embracing other aspects of staff management such as the skills of delegating work and of communicating with, motivating and supervising the staff.

Recruitment and interviewing of staff may be helped when *job descriptions* are prepared beforehand. These give a general description of the work which has to be done and maybe the type of person required to do it.

Specimen Job Description for a Floor Housekeeper

Job title	Floor Housekeeper.
Place of work	Woodlands Hotel. Housekeeping Department.
Purpose of job	1 To supervise Room-maids' and House-porters' work on an allocated number of floors and to ensure that work is carried out to the standard required by the Executive Housekeeper.
	2 To ensure that departure rooms are serviced and made ready as soon as possible in order that reception may re-let at any time.
	3 To anticipate the guests' requirements at all times thereby ensuring comfort and satisfaction.
Hours of work	7.30 a.m.–4.30 p.m. operated on a rota
	8.30 a.m.–5.30 p.m. system 5 days per
	2 p.m.–10 p.m. week.
Responsible to	Executive Housekeeper.

Responsible for	Room-maids, Houseporters, Cleaners, Cloak-room Attendants.
Liaison with	Receptionists, Head Floor Waiter, Valets, Linen Room Staff, Hall Porter and Store-keeper.
Scope of Work	Help with training of staff.
	Maintaining stocks.
	Maintaining set standards of work.
	Planning of work.
	Reporting to Executive Housekeeper or her deputy problems in carrying out the job.

Routine duties

1 Checking staff on duty.
2 Issuing keys.
3 Supervising room-maids, houseporters and cleaners.
4 Checking all rooms on floors.
5 Issuing cleaning stores.
6 Supervising linen requirements and checking floor stocks are correct.
7 Keeping in constant contact with reception.
8 Reporting maintenance work.
9 Attending to guests' requirements.
10 Reporting immediately to the Management and/or Security any persons who may be acting suspiciously.
11 Undertaking any job delegated by the Executive Housekeeper or her deputy.

Occasional duties

1 Supervising the changing of curtains, bedding, etc.
2 Attending staff meetings.
3 Further training of staff.
4 Dealing with simple first aid.
5 Helping with stocktaking.
6 Planning of extra work.
7 Attending fire drills.

Job procedures specify the way in which a job is to be done (order of work cards p. 42). They should be planned in relation to a specific establishment taking into account different surfaces, different cleaning equipment and agents, and should help in deciding the number of staff required and in training the staff in correct working methods. In addition they should be planned to:

aid standardisation;
preserve surfaces, materials;

effect a saving of cleaning equipment and agents;
effect a saving of employees' time;
effect a saving of employees' energy;
prevent accidents;
aid the compiling of work schedules.

Work schedules list the actual work to be undertaken by particular members of staff during a particular period of the day. Times of meals, breaks and any special jobs are pinpointed throughout the period so that there is a guide not only as to what has to be done but also when it has to be done. Order of work cards may supplement work schedules. Work schedules should be essentially simple in form with the minimum number of words and should be planned to:
make the best use of staff;
ensure coverage of work;
ensure fair allocation of work.

Specimen Work Schedule for Domestic Assistant in a hospital ward.

7.05 a.m.	Dust and vacuum sister's office
7.20	Vacuum wards and clean treatment room
8.30	Collect breakfast trays, waterjugs and glasses
9.00	Damp dust wards; replace locker bags. Return water jugs and glasses
9.45	Prepare trolley for coffee
10.00	Serve coffee
10.15	Coffee break
10.45	Collect coffee cups
11.00	Clean bathroom, sluices and lavatories
11.45	Thoroughly wash hands
	Lay table and trays for lunch
	Prepare kitchen for service
	Serve after lunch teas
	Clean kitchen
1.30 p.m.	Lunch
2.00	Extra work on regular days:
	wash bedtables
	wash wheel chairs
	wash flower vases
	polish furniture
	tidy and clean linen cupboard
	change curtains
3.00	Prepare and serve teas
	Collect trays
	Wash out cloths, put equipment away
3.55	Off duty

In order to enable the right member of staff to be on duty at the right time **duty rosters** are compiled. These should be clearly laid out showing the hours of duty and days off for each member of staff as well as any other relevant details such as mealtimes. (See p. 58.) They should be planned to:

enable areas to be covered for the correct periods;
see whether there is over or under staffing at any particular time;
ensure fair allocation of hours and days off.

As a manager, the *housekeeper leads and directs*; she gives instructions, trains and motivates her staff to meet the required standards. Incentive bonuses may be useful short term motivators but the *housekeeper* should look further than this. Good staff relations and good working conditions are probably longer term motivators. In planning well the *housekeeper* improves staff relationships and should at all times act as an example to her staff and provide them with the cohesive force of leadership and purpose. She should ensure discipline is kept at a reasonable level consistent with managerial policy and make her staff aware of the need to take their share in the efficient and economic running of the department. (See Chapter 1.)

Staff have more faith in the *housekeeper* who shows command of the situation and this applies not only to the usual work of organising the department but also to the way in which she deals with emergencies occurring from time to time. These emergencies could be, for example, fire, accident, death or birth and in all cases the *housekeeper* is expected to keep a cool head and to maintain discipline and control over staff and guests according to house policy.

Having selected her staff, the *housekeeper* should:

give them as good working conditions as possible;
see that they have the right 'tools' for the job;
train them for the job;
motivate them to the job;
supervise them on the job.

To ensure that everything works to give a balanced, effective organisation the *housekeeper* needs to *co-ordinate* the activities of the department. She should keep the department running smoothly, dealing with problems and queries as they arise, giving consideration to guest and staff welfare and maintaining liaison with other heads of departments (see Chapter 1). Effective means of communication are of vital importance.

In *controlling* her department, the *housekeeper* constantly checks performance and work results. This involves keeping an ever watchful eye on the work in progress and the costs incurred, and collecting information regarding the work from her assistants. Planning and control are complementary and where the *housekeeper* finds any deviation from the original plan she should take the necessary steps to remedy it, or she may consider it advisable to replan.

In aiming at an efficiently run department with as low operating costs as possible the *housekeeper* endeavours to save time, labour and materials. In doing so, she controls not only work methods, allocation of work and the working conditions of her staff but also all articles in use within the department, e.g. linen, uniforms, keys, furniture and furnishings, equipment and supplies, and ensures as far as she is able security (p. 235), the prevention of accidents (p. 239), the provision of first aid (p. 241) and the prevention of damage by insect or other pests (p. 246) throughout the department.

The *housekeeper* carries the direct responsibility for achieving the aims of her department and the only way she can have effective control is by close and careful supervision. While she delegates much of the routine work and day to day supervision of the department to her assistants she must remain observant and perceptive and be, at all times, someone to whom the staff can look up and turn for advice.

(N.B. In the smaller establishments the *housekeeper* is much more concerned with the day to day routine work and at times may have no assistants on duty with her.)

In surveying and controlling the work of her department, the *housekeeper* should keep abreast of new products, furnishings, uniforms, etc. and in doing so she should try out new materials, equipment, supplies and the like in an endeavour to keep costs as low as possible. New ideas may be gained by visiting exhibitions and other establishments, by reading trade magazines and by seeing representatives from the various firms when they call. These are all time consuming but essential if up-to-date products and methods etc. are to be used and operating costs kept down.

A **budget** is a plan of expenditure and if there is to be any control of costs throughout the establishment, budgeting is essential. The *housekeeper* is one of those concerned with the preparation of a budget for her department.

She estimates the expenditure for her department for a specified period; this is generally a year but there is at least one group of hotels where the *housekeeper* estimates on a monthly basis. The longer the financial period obviously the more difficult it is to forecast the requirements and relevant costs for the department.

There are three broad areas to be considered when preparing the budget:

wages and salaries,
operating costs (supplies, services, etc.),

capital expenditure (equipment usually with a life of 5 years or more or over a fixed sum of money).

The *housekeeper* should consider past records regarding occupancy rates, wages and salaries, purchases of equipment, furnishings, etc. in an endeavour to forecast future labour requirements, increases in wages, new services being planned, replacement of equipment, linen, furniture, furnishings, etc.

She should therefore include in her budget the probable cost of:

wages, salaries and contracts,
additional cleaning equipment, furniture, furnishings, etc.,
replacement of cleaning equipment and agents, guests' supplies, furniture, furnishings, linen, etc.,
repairs,
and in some cases, planned renovation and redecoration.

The *housekeeper* should realise that changes may occur in such external factors as the labour market, the commodity market and in legislation and these may all have a bearing on her estimation of the expenditure of the department over the next financial year.

The *housekeeper* should be preparing throughout the financial period for the presentation of the next budget by keeping records of relevant facts, e.g. the usage of various agents, the cost of repair services, etc. In this way she is more easily able to justify the cost of particular items. It is helpful if a priority rating is made for each item and if some indication is given as to whether an item is a replacement, an improvement or an addition. Higher priority ratings are normally given to replacements than to additions. Management requires to be furnished with records, observations and evaluations of past performance and plans for the future.

The *housekeeper* should offer advice (tactfully where not requested) on matters relating to the choice of floors and other finishes, furnishings, furniture and other fittings to ensure that due consideration is given to economy in cleaning.

An advantage in preparing a budget is that it provides the opportunity to take a critical look at the costs of the department, review past planning and present accomplishments and appropriate steps may then be taken to accomplish more in the coming financial period. In this connection it may be beneficial for the *housekeeper* to look more closely at the cost of such things as:

servicing of a room;
cleaning of a particular area;
serving of early morning teas;

night service, i.e. 'turning down';
overtime compared with extra staff;
hiring compared with owning linen;
checking of linen;
using non iron linen with or without laundry on premises;
office supplies, hand written versus duplicated versus printed lists;
re-upholstering versus purchasing new;
use of contracts;
bulk buying.

In some establishments direct labour may not always be the most suitable and the advisability of **contract arrangements** for cleaning may have to be considered by the *housekeeper*.

When choosing between contract and direct ('in-house') labour one is not only concerned with a comparison of cost, service and convenience but also with which will be best within the existing organisation of the establishment.

For example, in places where *housekeepers* are as yet not appointed, as is still the case in many hospitals and the administrative officer is more concerned with other problems, it would seem reasonable that contract labour might be an advantage. In other instances, due to the existence of a good housekeeping organisation contract labour might seem unnecessary, except perhaps for helping out with periodic and annual cleaning of particular areas. It is mainly in this field that hotels are employing contractors, e.g. for window cleaning, upholstery and carpet cleaning.

Basically the decision between contract and direct labour must be made on the amount of money available. It has been suggested that a contractor must be *20–30 per cent. more productive* than direct labour in order to provide an *equal service* at an *equal cost* and still get a fair profit.

Window cleaning was the first service to be offered on a contract basis, but now general and specialised cleaning is being undertaken in all types of establishments.

A typical contract cleaning firm may offer a wide range of services amongst which will be:

complete cleaning programmes with all work and responsibility undertaken by the contractor;
selected types of cleaning within the establishments, e.g. the cleaning of particular areas, night cleaning, etc.;
periodic services to assist the existing housekeeping organisation, e.g. window cleaning, wall washing, carpet and upholstery cleaning.

The main advantages of contract labour to the client are:

there is no capital outlay for equipment;

there is no equipment (particularly specialised equipment) lying idle;

the difficulty of finding, training, organising and supervising the cleaning staff is passed to the contractor;

extra work may be carried out at certain times without increasing the basic staff;

the exact cost of cleaning is known for a given period.

With a good contractor it is possible that a higher level of cleanliness at the same cost may be obtained because of new methods and more efficient equipment and materials being used. Materials will be bought in large quantities and so may be bought more cheaply and this may be reflected in the cost of the service. (Although these represent only a small proportion—possibly 5–10 per cent.—of the total cost of any cleaning process.)

In spite of these advantages there are many dissatisfied clients and many of them have reverted to direct labour.

Causes of dissatisfaction may be:

loss of flexibility to effect changes;

loss of proprietary interest. The cleaners do not belong to, i.e. do not work for, the establishment;

problems regarding security;

problems regarding liaison and co-operation between departments;

deterioration in the quality of the work. One of the reasons for this may be the great growth of contract firms over the last few years, resulting in cut price tenders being offered and accepted (clients almost always accept the lowest price) which do not enable contractors to employ a sufficient number of employees or employees of the right calibre to do the job properly. Supervision is all important and the right supervisor essential; good workers should be the result of good supervision.

Deterioration in the quality of the work may not always be the fault of the contractor; it may be that the client has not fully understood the contract. (The cleaner will not lift the mats unless it says so in the schedule.) It is essential that a specific contract is drawn up, outlining the responsibilities of both parties and in this way, both the client and the contractor know what is expected of the other and a dangerous cause of potential dissatisfaction is removed.

Specifications should therefore be carefully worded and may cover the following points:

the frequency with which a job is to be done—5/6/7 days a week, once or twice a day, etc.;

the hours during which work is to be done;

security requirements (sometimes all staff are 'vetted' and all specified rooms have to be kept locked);

adequate supervisory requirements;

storage areas and provision of lockers and other accommodation for the staff;

inspections with client;

regular meetings with the client;

public and customer liability (insurance).

The contract itself will state the duration of contract, the price for the job and whether an initial clean is required before the contract comes into operation.

Most contracts are agreed on a unit rate agreement. The *housekeeper* provides details of the area and the frequency and asks how much. The reliable contractor measures and calculates the cost.

Man hours = Areas to be covered x time allowed x frequency

To the cost of wages (operators and supervision) he adds cost of equipment, agents and supplies, overheads and profit.

The contractor who wants the job often guesses the lowest price and the contract invariably goes to the lowest bidder who may have to cut standards to cover his losses.

A far better contract than one agreed on a unit cost basis is one where the contractor is reimbursed for the costs of the job and given a fixed fee. In this case, there is no point in his cutting his cost because he has a guaranteed profit. A one-year contract basis is thought to be unsatisfactory; a three or five year contract is better and the costs should be escalating over the period.

With the costs plus fixed fee type of contract, the *housekeeper* specifies staff and equipment etc. Specifications for a contractor should be the same as for direct or 'in-house' labour and the *housekeeper* should calculate cleaning costs from cost of wages, equipment, agents and supplies.

e.g. 400 hours per week at 60p an hour   = £14,480 per year
      Supervision   1,500
      Small equipment and supplies (cloths, etc.)   275
      Capital equipment (written off over 10 years)

10 vacuum cleaners	£600
1 polisher	£100
1 scrubber	£100
2 dustettes	£40
	£840

Capital investment over 10 years   84
Cleaning agents   325
    Total cleaning cost per year is £16,664

This can be expressed as cost per square metre if required.

Besides contract cleaning other contract arrangements may be made by the *housekeeper* for her department with:

a laundry—when a price is approved by weight or per flat article provided a minimum number is sent;

a florist—when an agreement is made to provide floral arrangements for specific areas over a given period at a specified price;

various manufacturing firms for the

servicing of equipment at stated intervals;

delivery of certain goods at stated intervals;

various hire firms

linen (p. 86).

equipment (p. 22).

furniture and furnishings (p. 193).

In the case of equipment, furniture and furnishings the contract is made for a given number of years, after which a new contract for new articles may be made or the old articles may be retained at a reduced price. Leasing contracts for hard furniture and upholstery in leather or expanded vinyl are generally written over a 5-7 year lease period while those for soft furnishings are for a shorter period, generally 3 years.

At the end of the primary leasing period when a new contract for new articles is written it is usual for a 'trade-in' allowance to be given, equal to the residual value of the original items.

In all cases it is necessary to pay great attention to the terms of the lease and to use firms of good repute. Leasing does however mean no capital outlay, budgeting is made easier because costs are known and it is possible to modernise immediately and pay for the modernisation with future profits.

When **buying** on a large scale many aspects must be considered and the amount of money available plays an important part. The actual buying may be done by a specific buyer, the manager of an hotel or the *housekeeper*. Where the establishment belongs to a group the buying may be done centrally, and the items are then ordered from the central office and these may include floorings, furniture, soft furnishings, linen, crockery, equipment, etc.

Goods may be bought direct from the manufacturers (in which case there may be a minimum stipulated), from a wholesaler or from a retailer. Much useful information regarding new products and new methods may be obtained by seeing representatives, always remembering that in many cases their livelihood depends on the orders that they get. In any case the source should be a reputable one in order that complaints and discrepancies will receive attention.

Before buying the following general points should be considered:

Are the items really necessary?
What wear and tear will they be subjected to?
How easily are they cleaned?
How easily are they maintained?
What is the minimum quantity necessary?
What materials and designs will suit the purpose?
What colour, pattern and texture will fit in with the general scheme?

When consideration has been given to the above, specifications should be drawn up and firms asked to submit quotations by a certain date. Quotations outside the proposed price range should be rejected and the other firms asked to submit samples. These should be tested and discussion regarding pattern, quantities, special marking (badging or cresting) and final price should take place.

Where appropriate, colours should be seen in natural and artificial light and due consideration given to wastage of material where large patterns are used for fabrics, carpets and wall coverings.

Standardisation may lead to a saving in money because articles may be interchanged and less stock required, especially for crockery. Further saving in money may be possible by buying one large quantity at one time rather than several small amounts as a better discount may often be obtained. Against this, capital is lying idle and so, when buying, the availability and the notice required for replacements should be considered. The buying of cleaning agents and in particular buying in bulk versus individual packs has been mentioned in Chapter 2 (p. 38). Stock books and monthly consumption sheets are a guide when re-ordering consumable goods as quantities used in a given period are then known. Standing orders are sometimes given for certain articles but these can lead to over or under stocking and may mean that advantage cannot be taken of good offers.

All goods should be checked on arrival for quantity, quality and condition since the sooner complaints are made, the better attention they will receive.

Specimen specification for a carpet
Constructional requirements

Construction	Wilton
No. of colours	2
Composition of surface yarn	80%/20% Wool/BriNylon
Height of pile (above backing)	10 mm.
Backing material	cotton/jute

Performance requirements
The materials will be subjected to a number of tests including:

Dynamic loading B.S.4052—loss of pile height after 1,000 impacts not more than 30%.
Compression recovery B.S.4098—recovery not less than 80%.

Results of tests

Sample	No. of rubs	% compression recovery	% loss in pile height	pile weight	Composition		
					Wool	nylon	Price
1	100,000	78.9	9.8	1,722	71.5	28.5	£5.05
2	44,000	67.8	15.8	811	72.7	27.3	4.10
3	90,000	73.8	16.1	1,187	77.7	22.3	4.75

The keeping of records

Paper work is necessary and although time consuming the *housekeeper* will need to keep certain records in order to aid memory, to improve efficiency and to make it easier should someone have to take over her job. Not all records are relevant to all types of establishments, but amongst those kept may be:

  records of recruitment for staff and their results;
  records of staff, giving personal particulars, e.g. date of commencement of employment, next of kin, holidays, sickness, absences, date of leaving with reasons and possibly brief notes on their work and conduct in case of requests for references;
  record of hours worked by staff;
  record of staff training;
  stock books for linen and stores;
  inventories of furniture and equipment, dates of receipt, cost and possibly record of maintenance;
  records of each room regarding redecoration, new furnishings and annual cleaning;
  blanket book;
  lost property book;
  accident book;
  record of individual personal tastes of frequent guests and V.I.P.'s;
  financial records—costs of personnel, room servicing, cleaning, contracts, purchasing of equipment and supplies, etc.

Communications

In any establishment there are times when staff and *guests* need to be contacted and unless there is a good system of communication tempers may become frayed, and time and energy wasted. Communications may be required between *guest* and staff, staff and staff and *guest* and *guest*, when the giving and receiving of information, instructions and complaints as well as the dealing with requests and emergencies may take place.

The telephone system is probably the most used means of communication and apart from 'memos' the only form for *guest* to *guest*. The larger the number of instruments strategically placed the more effective but more costly the system will be. (There are hotels where telephones are installed in private bathrooms and even some where there are two instruments provided in double bedrooms.) Contact may be made by direct dialling or through the switchboard operator. Where dialling is direct the calls may be internal or external and in the latter case in hotels, the charges are 'clocked' up automatically to the occupant of the room. (It would appear that in this case there is no measure of control over the misuse of the telephone by unauthorised persons. The meter is normally only read on the departure of the guest.)

Telephones can lead to many interruptions and where messages are being received continuously it may be convenient to have them recorded on tape, when they may be played back as required. In hotels messages between the housekeeper and the receptionist, the guest and the valet, etc., may be recorded in this way. An electro-writer may also be used between one department and another when the machine transmits and records hand written messages.

Different coloured lights or a combination of coloured lights indicate on a room status board to the receptionist and the housekeeper the state of the rooms, i.e. whether the rooms are vacated, being serviced or ready. When a guest has paid his bill the light is operated by the receptionist or cashier and first the maid and then the housekeeper override this light with a 'jack' placed in a socket in the guest's room. In new large hotels this system is computerised; there is then only one light by the side of each room number on the board and by pressing the appropriate button e.g. rooms being serviced, the receptionist or housekeeper can obtain the necessary information regarding the rooms. A small light by the telephone in his room may indicate to the guest that a message is waiting at reception.

Two-way communication is possible in some places where a master console unit is to be found in some convenient place—Sister's office in a nursing home or hospital, reception in an hotel, and a small cabinet is in the patient's or guest's room. In some hotels there is an intercom-cum-baby listener.

In many old buildings press buttons in rooms or by beds in hospitals and nursing homes operate lights or bells in convenient places (e.g. corridors, service rooms, etc.), indicating that a particular service is required. At one time there was always a bellpush in hotel bathrooms, but in many new buildings this is no longer the case. Except where there is a telephone within easy reach this would appear to be a retrograde step as accidents and emergencies do occur in bathrooms. A bell system is, of course, used to raise the alarm in the case of fire or a breakdown in lifts and fire alarms may be connected direct to the fire station.

Paging systems are other means of communication and only in luxury hotels are there page boys or messengers. Public address systems are still used in some establishments but these can prove disturbing. The 'bleep' is a limited paging system; in this case certain members of staff whose work takes them all over the establishment, and the *housekeeper* is one such person, carry a small battery operated device which 'bleeps' when the particular person is required. It is worked via the switchboard and the member of staff 'bleeped' goes to a telephone to find out why he or she is wanted.

Memoranda are means of leaving messages for a person, or of confirming some verbal communication. The visual communication is often better than the verbal one and in hotels there are many, e.g. arrival and departure lists, room occupancy lists, slept outs, early morning tea lists, etc. These communications are between department and department, but in addition there are communications found in hotel bedrooms, designed to be informative in order that the guest may use the services of the hotel to his/her advantage. A folder containing such communications as 'Do not disturb', 'Please clean my room', 'Room service order', 'Directory of services', 'Laundry and valeting service and price list' can prove extremely useful to the guest and save the staff a great deal of time.

While communications are not a 'tool' of management, good communications are essential for the smooth running of all establishments and so any person in a managerial position, such as the *housekeeper*, is as concerned with communications as she is with the engagement and welfare of her staff, the planning, organisation, budgeting and the economic running of her department.

Glossary

Architraves are the mouldings round doors and windows.

Bedding is the term used for the articles on a bed, and normally includes the launderable linen.

Block Tips are a share of tips, usually from tours, conferences, etc., which the *housekeeper* distributes with discretion, amongst her staff.

Cantilevered refers to articles resting on a bracket projecting from a wall.

Ceramics are articles made from clay, e.g. china and tiles.

Checkout is the American term for a departure in an hotel.

Cleaning Agents or Materials include abrasives, detergents, solvents, polishes, etc.

Cleaning Equipment includes brooms and brushes, electrical equipment, containers, cleaning cloths, etc.

Cutlery loosely embraces spoons, forks as well as knives.

Departure is a room from which a guest is expected to leave or has already left.

Discards are condemned articles in the linen room which may be renovated for other uses or used as rag.

Ergonomics is the study of mankind in relation to his working environment.

Floor Seals are semi-permanent finishes of cellulosic or plastic composition, applied to render a floor impermeable and to protect its surface.

Furnishings include soft furnishings, carpets and furniture.

General Assistant is a person who in a small hotel assists generally in any department.

In situ means 'on the spot' or 'on site'.

Linen is a material woven from flax, but the term 'linen' is often used loosely, to denote launderable articles found in the linen room.

OOO—out of order.

Ready room is one which has been serviced and is ready for re-letting.

Refurbish is to give a 'new look' to a room by redecorating, the renewing of soft furnishings and possibly the carpet, and the 'touching up' of furniture.

Re-sheeting means putting out clean towels in a bedroom and making up the beds with clean sheets and slips.

Room State or Occupancy List is the list on which the maid states whether the room is vacant or occupied and, if possible, the number of sleepers in each room, and it is required by the receptionist and control office in a large hotel, at regular times each day.

Soft Furnishings include curtains, cushions, loose covers, bedspreads and quilts, but not carpets.

Spread-over is the total number of hours over which a duty extends in any one day, e.g. 7 a.m.–2 p.m. and 6–10 p.m. has a spread-over of 15 hours.

Textiles are woven fabrics, e.g. cotton sheeting.

Turning Down is the term applied to the work maids do each evening in guests' bedrooms in hotels.

Uniform is a 'dress' of specified material, colour and design, usually provided by the establishment for certain staff.

Vacant room is one previously serviced and not yet occupied.

Vacated room is one from which the guest has left.

Index